Creating Life Against The Odds

Creating Life Against The Odds

The Journey From Infertility To Parenthood

Ilona Laszlo Higgins MD, FACOG

Copyright © 2006 by Ilona Laszlo Higgins MD, FACOG

Library of Congress Control Number:		2006907633
ISBN 10:	Hardcover	1-4257-3067-1
	Softcover	1-4257-3066-3
ISBN 13:	Hardcover	978-1-4257-3067-3
	Softcover	978-1-4257-3066-6

All rights reserved. No part of this book may be reproduced or transmitted in any form or by any means, electronic or mechanical, including photocopying, recording, or by any information storage and retrieval system, without permission in writing from the copyright owner.

This book was printed in the United States of America.

To order additional copies of this book, contact:
Xlibris Corporation
1-888-795-4274
www.Xlibris.com
Orders@Xlibris.com
36102

This book is dedicated to my children, Dauber, Jessica, and Tucker, who have made my life a joy, and to my husband, David, who has made it an adventure.

CONTENTS

Acknowledgments 13
Foreword 15
Introduction 19

Chapter 1: Starting the Journey 25
    Don't Try to Go It Alone: The Need for
        Emotional Reinforcement
    Identifying Infertility
    Who are the Infertile?
    When to Seek Help Getting Pregnant
    Who's your Doctor? Ob/Gyn vs. Specialist
    Are You Ready for ART?
    The Unknowns with ART

Chapter 2: When the Heart Calls: Battling Infertility 45
    Facing the Emptiness: Dealing with Yourself
    Fielding Feedback: Dealing with Outsiders
    Keeping the Dream Alive
    Riding the Emotional Roller Coaster:
        How to Support your Partner
    Reality Check: The Financial Costs
    Handling It Together
    And Now the Wait
    It Takes Two
    A Word about Intimacy
    Another Happy Ending

Chapter 3: The World of Assisted Reproductive
             Technology (ART) 63
   The Birth Matrix: An Illustrated Guide to All the Options
   My Story: A Rocky Start
   The Secrecy Issue: Do You Want to Know your Donor?
   When One Door Closes, Another Opens
   My Story Continues: A Surprise and a Tough Choice
   Katie's Boys
   Message to ART Professionals: What We Need to Do
       Differently
   A Tale of Two Consults

Chapter 4: Gifts From the Heart: The Other Partners
             in Your ART Experience 91
   Sperm and Egg Donation
   Who is the Parent? Psychological and Legal Issues
       Justina and Mark: Using a Gestational Carrier
       Elaine and Arthur: Using an Ovum Donor
       Arlene and Faith: Using Both Ovum and Sperm
           Donors
   The Hearts and Minds of the Donors
       Mariah, Ovum Donor: A Big Honor for a Small Role
       Jori, Ovum Donor: Passing on Special Qualities
       Rose-Marie, Ovum Donor: Influenced by Adoption
       Melinda, Ovum Donor: Inspired by Nature
       Peter, Sperm Donor: Touched by Tragedy
       Kami and Sam, Embryo Donors: Sharing the Bounty
   Receiving Donor Genes and Mourning the Lost Genetic
       Link
   Fathers and Donor Sperm
   On Using a Sperm Donor: Who's the Real Daddy?
   Mothers and Donor Sperm
   Fathers and Donor Ovum
   Mothers and Donor Ovum

Considerations When Choosing a Donor
The Donor-Recipient Contract
The Confidentiality Questions:
> Do You Want to Know your Donor?
> Should You be Open about Using ART?
>> Bernadette: Still Undecided
>> Kendra: Single Mom
>> Irina: Religious and Ethnic Considerations
>> Krista: Responding Creatively to Friends
>> Annabelle: Feeling Isolated by Secrecy
>> Katerina: Protecting her Child's Privacy
>> Christina: Telling Only Those Who've Had the Experience

A Lesson of History—and Secrecy
Messages to Give Yourself

Chapter 5: The Surrogate Experience 127
Selecting a Surrogate
A Tale of Two Surrogates
The Womb Connection
What is a Parent? A Global Perspective
Bearing Her Sister's Baby
No Greater Gift

Chapter 6: Pregnant at Last! 141
My Story: Facing the Unexpected
My Story: Further Complications
The Legacy of Infertility
Other Emotional Repercussions
Prenatal Care and Confidentiality
The Little Stranger Inside
The Magic Moment: Delivery
My Story: Dauber, Jessica, and Tucker
A Lesson in Etiquette

Chapter 7: Bringing Baby Home **161**
- The Ties that Bind
    - Marsha: Learning about Patience and Trust
    - Ginny: Instant Bonding
    - Pamela: Mom by Adoption and by Ovum Donation
    - Holly: Tying the Apron Strings
    - My Story: Sharing Tucker with Jessica
- The Solomon Syndrome
- Post Partum Depression
    - My Story: Depression and Recovery
- The Reality of Parenthood
    - Hillary: "Don't Over Analyze"
    - Remi: Thoughts on Genetics
    - Melanie: The Irony of Looks
    - Rhonda: Seeing her Donor in her Son
    - Megan: Finding Completion
    - Bette: It's the Commitment that Counts
    - Marlene: A Special Farewell

Chapter 8: Telling Children Their Stories **177**
- Finding the Way
- The Rewards of Openness
- My Story: How I Told Tucker
- Tailoring Your Tale
    - Nancy: What a Five-Year-Old Tells her Best Friend
    - Miranda: Wizards and Magic Brews
    - Meredith: Four Little Girls and Three Ways to Make a Family
    - Kitt: Making Eggs Out of Clay
    - Coleen: Sperms, Worms, and Germs
- As Time Goes By
- In Their Own Words

    Fifteen-Year-Old Ken Talks about his Origins
    Twelve-Year-Old Tally on Understanding her Dad
    Seventeen-Year-Old Kela: Forever Grateful to her Adoptive Parents
    Fourteen-Year-Old Ryan on the Importance of Honesty
    "The Return" by Theresa Tanner
  Letting Love Multiply

Afterword 199

Appendix I: Basic Facts about Infertility 201
    Common Causes of Female Infertility
    Common Causes of Male Infertility

Appendix II: What To Expect: Common Tests and Procedures 207

Appendix III: Ethics and Embryos 213
    Is Parenthood a Person's Right?
    Are Doctors Obliged to Help the Infertile?
    Is IVF Ethically or Morally Wrong?
    What about the Selecting of Some Embryos for Transfer while Rejecting Others?
    Is there a Risk of People Trying for "Designer Babies?"
    Who is the "Real Parent" of an IVF Child?
    Is the Compensation of Donors Unethical?
    Ethics and Politics

Appendix IV: Avoiding Missteps and Misdirection: Problems with Language 229

Acknowledgments

Thank you to Phyllis Wender for believing in me right from the start, to Lee Quarfoot for keeping after me to find clarity of voice, and to Amanda Mecke for trying to get the publishing establishment to take on this sensitive subject matter.

Thank you to my medical colleagues: Amos Madanes, Chris Northrup, and Richard Fisher, for their support and encouragement; Ralph Hale, who read every word more than once with infinite patience; Christos Coutifaris, for his many insightful recommendations; and Jack McDermott, psychiatrist and friend, who gave me that final read when the trees were all I could see of the forest.

Thank you to my mental health colleagues: Elizabeth Grill and Judith Kottick, whose insights into the experiences of fathers are, I hope, reflected in what I have to say to "dad;" and Carole Lieber Wilkins, who gave me new insights into disclosure issues, which she has examined with great sensitivity through both a professional as well as a parental lens.

Thank you to Mahlon Hoagland for helping to refine my understanding of genetics and to Kale Langlas for his comments on my description of hanai families in traditional Hawaiian culture.

A special thank you to my husband, David, for his patience and support, for his comments and suggestions, and for his help on Appendix III.

And finally, my deepest appreciation goes to all the parents, children, and donors who have so generously shared their stories with me over these past eight years. They are my heroes.

Ilona Higgins
Kamuela, Hawaii
August, 2006

Foreword

Attempting to achieve a pregnancy and failing can have devastating emotional effects upon a woman. Today's media has indoctrinated our culture to the point where failure to conceive is a failure as a woman. Fortunately, today modern pharmacology and technology have developed methods and procedures that give many more options. The uses of ovulation induction and assisted reproductive technology have allowed previously infertile couples to become pregnant and share the joys of parenthood. However, there are still those women who, for one or more reasons, fail to achieve a pregnancy with modern medications and technology. For those women, a variety of options are now available.

Dr. Ilona Higgins has addressed all of these issues in her book, *Creating Life Against the Odds*. Had this book been published 100 years ago or even 50 years ago, it would have been viewed as science fiction. At that time, science and medicine could not envision such far-reaching inroads into the arena of infertility. Today we take this for granted. However, this is the scientific view. What is the personal view of the patient and her family? It is this aspect that is so brilliantly explained in this book. The process of selection, fertilization, pregnancy, and delivery has been taken out of the arena of science and into the realm of everyday life.

Chapter One begins an exciting journey into the world of emotions and the unknown aspects of infertility and its treatment. It is presented by one who has been there and has faced the issues as a woman, not just as an obstetrician. Her personal insight is really expanded and presented in Chapter Two. The issue of the emotional "roller coaster" and need for support has never been presented so succinctly. When success occurs, it is worth the journey, but that is retrospective, and Dr. Higgins presents the everyday experience when the outcome is unknown.

The following chapters explore the world of assisted reproductive technology and its secrets. She shares deep personal revelations from her own experience, and she shares the experiences of other women who have gone through or are involved in the same procedures. Most inspiring is her description of the surrogate experience in Chapter Five. This is a subject seldom discussed in other publications, and Dr. Higgins explores it from the point of view of both parent and surrogate. The unique relationships that are forged through surrogacy are described with sensitivity by the author. This is difficult, emotional material that is very well presented.

The author then proceeds to explain pregnancy in her personal, nonscientific way, not as many books tend to explain it. Her exploration of the emotional aspects of pregnancy and delivery are most revealing and heart warming. There is the going home period and the adjustments that need to be made. There is even information on postpartum depression. This is an excellent addition and should give any new parent needed insight into the condition. The fact that a knowledgeable obstetrician could experience depression should help all women understand that this is a real phenomenon that should be discussed with their physicians and not something to hide.

The book ends with an excellent chapter on how to involve the family. Family involvement is key to any successful story, and her explanation is a guide to one way to succeed. Finally, the appendices are very helpful in describing and explaining the various components of assisted reproductive technology. Rather than being presented as a glossary, the question and answer or narrative format is much easier to understand.

For anyone who is contemplating any of the various methods of assisted reproductive technology, this book is a "gold mine" of helpful information. For those who are candidates for surrogate procedures, it is essential.

Ralph W. Hale, MD, FACOG
Executive Vice President
American College of Obstetricians and Gynecologists

Introduction

For more than 25 years, I've been honored to serve women of all ages, in many parts of the world, as an obstetrician/gynecologist. Along the way, I've counseled scores of infertile couples as they struggled to conceive, carry, and deliver a baby. In recent years, I have seen an increase in the number of couples seeking help, and I know that in the United States alone, more than 1.5 million couples use Assisted Reproductive Technology (ART) every year. In many of these cases, fertility treatment will require third party assistance in the form of donated germ cells (ova or sperm) or gestational care (surrogacy). When ART includes this kind of additional assistance, the process can be intense, exhausting—even debilitating. Most patients have no idea, starting out, of the emotional, spiritual, and ethical dilemmas they'll face, or the number of wrenching decisions they'll have to make.

Things weren't always so complicated, of course. Just a couple of generations ago, a baby's conception occurred only through the sexual union of a man and woman, and every baby was born carrying the genes of the birth mother and her mate. But today, a new life can begin outside the body, in vitro, with donated sperm and/or ova (eggs). A woman can carry a baby that does not share a genetic relationship with her or her partner.

The field of ART has made this all possible, providing unique opportunities for the conception and gestation of life. Someone going through the process may feel that little about it seems natural or normal. Yet I believe it's very important, as we embrace these new technologies, to remember that the fundamentals of pregnancy, birth, and a baby's needs, both before and after delivery, are the same everywhere on the planet.

As engaged as I was with the infertile couples in my medical practice, it wasn't until 1995 that I received an insider's look at the experience of ART. In that year, I myself sought out the help of ART. It was, to say the least, an eye-opening experience. I was 48, with a son and daughter who were nearly grown, and I suddenly, desperately, wanted another child. The realization startled me at first—and totally astounded my husband. But he saw the ardency of my need, and he quickly embraced the idea of being a dad one more time.

Our decision was made. But because of my age, the process wouldn't be a simple one. At 48, I had to accept that my eggs were unlikely to be viable. If we were going to have a chance for success, we would need to go the route of ovum donation, with the ovum to be fertilized, in vitro, with my husband's sperm.

My decision to become a mother again was made with the confidence of someone who was both a physician and a parent. But shortly after embarking on the ART journey, I made a sobering discovery. Despite my medical and parental expertise, I was totally unprepared for the consequences of my decision. I'd had no idea that I would face a profusion of fears and insecurities, both during my pregnancy and after the birth of my son.

How unique, I wondered, was my experience? I began to look around, on-line and in books and magazines, for stories of women who were trying to conceive or had recently been through assisted reproductive technologies similar to mine. I found thousands, and over the next few years I talked or corresponded with hundreds of them, focusing on the emotional impact of their decision to use ART. I learned, to my dismay, that many of them, like me, had marched through the doors of their infertility specialist's office psychologically unprepared for what they would encounter.

It is for all of these women, and for those who will follow in their footsteps, that I have written this book.

My own story—at least the part of it that shaped my thinking about parenthood and reproductive medicine—began one stormy night in December 1979. That was the night my husband, David, and I took a big step off our traditional New England career and life paths. A few months before, I had completed my residency at a Boston area hospital and had realized that I was no longer willing to maintain the 100-hour work weeks that had strained our marriage and had made it almost impossible to juggle my responsibilities as a physician and as the mother of two small children, ages six and one. David, meanwhile, had decided that he needed a break from the pressures and demands of his law practice in the corporate department of a large Boston law firm. The shared realization that we needed to make some big changes in our lives led us to sell our house, our two cars, and most of our personal possessions and to buy *Deliverance*, an 82-foot gaff schooner that we found tied up in the mangroves of English Harbour in Antigua. Our plan was to sail the oceans for 18 months while we sorted out what to do next.

We took *Deliverance* to Southwest Harbor, Maine for a six-month refit, and then we returned to Boston to say goodbye to family and friends. By late December, we were ready to set off. As we passed Minot's Light and watched the receding skyline of night-time Boston disappear into a swirl of snow, we began a journey that was to last for five magical years. *Deliverance* became our home, and I became a doctor-at-sea, providing emergency medical services and basic maternal and child health care to remote island communities, first in the Caribbean, and then throughout the Pacific. While our children were home schooled with the world as their classroom, my own education continued as I worked with midwives, traditional healers, and health assistants in different island cultures. I volunteered in hospitals in St. Lucia and Puerto Rico. I made medical rounds by dugout canoe in Roatan, Honduras. I was invited to participate in secret puberty rites ceremonies in the San Blas Islands in Panama. I learned new techniques for breech deliveries as a Senior Registrar in Ob/Gyn at National Women's Hospital in Auckland, New Zealand. And I did surgery by Coleman lantern in Papua New Guinea and on remote coral atolls in Micronesia.

In 1984, we finally settled in Hawaii, where I joined the faculty at the University of Hawaii's John A. Burns School of Medicine. As Assistant Director of Perinatal Services, I managed high-risk obstetrical referrals from all over the islands. At the same time, David and I maintained our commitment to the isolated island communities of Micronesia by founding a medical, non-profit service organization, Marimed Foundation. We frequently traveled with teams of volunteer doctors, nurses, and health educators between Hawaii and the Marshall Islands conducting clinics, and we made numerous trips to the U.S. Mainland, Japan, and Europe to raise funds to build a ship that would carry these volunteer health teams regularly to remote outer atoll communities that were without airstrips, electricity or plumbing. When the ship, *Tole Mour* (meaning "Gift of Life and Health" in the Marshallese language), went into service in 1988, our family lived on board, part of a floating community of nearly 50 volunteer doctors, dentists, nurses, and ship's crew. For nearly a year, I served as the project's Medical Director, and David was the ship's captain. Then, with mixed feelings, I turned over my responsibilities to another physician and started a private medical practice in Hawaii.

A very short six years later, our children were young adults, ready to leave home. The prospect of the empty-nest hit me hard. My years in academic medicine and private practice in Hawaii had been busy and fulfilling, but I realized that I had been overextended, often putting the needs of my career and my patients ahead of the needs of my children. I missed the magic of the six years we lived and traveled together as a family on *Deliverance* and *Tole Mour*, home-schooling the children. I realized that I wanted a chance to be a mother again, this time without the distraction of a demanding career. I wanted to extend the parenting chapter in my life and to expand the circle of love in our family. I believed the joy of a baby, a new sibling for our older children, would draw our older children back to the hearth. We'd have many new opportunities to be together again, but without the needs of the world taking precedence over our own.

In December of 1995, I learned I was pregnant with a donor egg and my husband's sperm. (More about my donor and my experience later on.) We were delighted that our plan was working. But during the latter half of the pregnancy, I found myself bombarded by confusing thoughts and feelings. "If this baby doesn't carry my genes," these thoughts said, "how can you be its mother? What have you gotten yourself into?" I was shocked at myself because these thoughts sharply contradicted my personal convictions. My experiences as a doctor and my exposure to so many different cultures had shown me repeatedly that mothering is much more than genes. Nature and nurture, I believed, were not factors that existed on opposite ends of a spectrum, but were woven together tighter than a tatami mat. Yet, from the perspective of this pregnancy, the weave was difficult for me to distinguish and understand.

After my son was born and I looked into his eyes, I found myself doubting that I was worthy to be the mother of such a precious treasure. Had I been fair, I wondered, to the rest of my family? Was I guilty for having done something based on my own needs rather than those of others? What had I wrought? And what about the future? Most children eventually take an interest in learning how they happened to be born. How and when was I going to communicate the details to my child? How could I insure his emotional and psychological well-being?

In time, I found my answers to these questions, just as other ART parents have resolved similar issues that confronted them. Raising an ART child has been a complicated challenge for many of us. Often, we've felt alone in our struggle. The field of ART has advanced so fast, it has exceeded our culture's capacity to integrate it. Families, friends and communities, no matter how well meaning, may not be equipped to offer adequate support.

In isolation, without a clear sense of shared pride in the immense journey they have undertaken to create their children, many ART parents find their confidence shaken. In the pages that follow, I have tried to explore in detail all the complex issues that can arise in the process—so that ART parents can decide for themselves how to proceed, and so that they can happily raise a generation of self-confident children.

Chapter 1

Starting the Journey

Katherine came into my office and dropped heavily into the wide wicker chair beside my desk. She was glowing. After nine years of trying to become pregnant, she was due to deliver a healthy baby girl in two weeks, conceived with her husband's sperm and a donated ovum.

"I can see that you're enjoying every moment," I told her. "It's what you deserve. You've both been through so much and have finally emerged victorious."

"Sometimes I do feel like the heroine of my own adventure story," she answered. "I had to fight for my baby, and there were terrible obstacles at every step."

"But it was all worth it?" I asked, although I knew the answer. "You'd encourage other women to take the plunge?"

"Sure," she said, "but I'd warn them that they'd be crossing the borders of the known world into a strange land, and they'd have to be ready to do battle."

"What else would you tell them?"

Katherine paused. "I'd tell them that disasters and setbacks are a normal part of the experience," she said, "that there may be egg or sperm donors who drop out, needles to face, doctors with bad attitudes, and your own body saying 'no,' but you have to stand up and be fierce. You will have to go to the darkest abyss in search of your child, and you need to be mighty, to arm yourself with courage. And, God willing, you will get that child and return to the normal world, stronger than before. Maybe that child will be, in part, from another woman's ovum, or be carried by someone else, but it is yours. You fought for that child's life. You brought it into the world."

Katherine hit the nail on the head. Assisted reproduction is not for the meek. That doesn't mean that to be successful one must consider the experience akin to a battle-ground; not everyone does. But most would agree there are many unknowns when you enter the world of assisted reproductive technologies seeking to conceive a child. Some of us feel less like confident warriors and more like exhausted swimmers being carried along by a tide of procedures, and we're not always sure whether the tide, in the end, will carry us to a happy and safe shore or just further out to sea.

Of course, life always throws challenges at us. If we're lucky, these help us to mature and know ourselves better. But, sometimes, when confronted with infertility, we may discover that we don't know ourselves so well after all.

Infertility can be a nasty surprise, especially for a woman who has never questioned her body's ability to perform natural functions. It creates self-doubt, guilt, depression, even self-blame. It raises bitter questions: Why can't I have a baby? Did I do something wrong? Am I being punished? At a time when we least expect it, in our otherwise most productive years, we're forced to revisit issues we confronted as teenagers, to ask again: Who am I? Where am I going? What's my purpose in life?

As Katherine said, infertility can be one of life's greatest challenges. And like any challenge we face, it can bring out the best in us. It can reveal our strength and resilience and help us identify our priorities. But it can also bring out our darkest nature and leave us shattered and devastated, with broken marriages and broken hearts. Couples may experience years of frustration, spend tens of thousands of dollars, and be compelled to accept compromises they never imagined. And no matter how infertility is ultimately resolved—through ART, adoption, or the decision to live child-free—it can leave a haunting legacy.

The challenge doesn't end if a woman becomes pregnant. She may feel anxiety during the months she's waiting for her baby to be born. Sometimes the aftermath of her former barrenness is a feeling of unworthiness that's similar to survivor's guilt. She wonders whether she deserves to be a mother. She fears her child will be taken away by some cruel fate, long after delivery.

Individuals or couples who decide to undertake any form of ART are pioneers, out there on one of science's frontiers, without the comfort that comes from decades of historical perspective, and the experience can feel very isolating. They come to their high-tech parenthood weary and depleted, having suffered major doubts about their self-worth and role in the world. But because they made difficult choices and were tested in ways no parent of a spontaneously conceived child could imagine, they may also have discovered the fortitude and wisdom to be exceptionally fine parents.

Don't Try to Go It Alone: The Need for Emotional Reinforcement

Being a pioneer means that there may not be readily available support along the way. When you are infertile, you can't rely on the fertile world to be helpful or understanding. Even within the medical profession, I'm sorry to say, empathy and guidance can be in short supply.

One of the most disturbing comments that I've heard from time to time from colleagues is that it might just be "God's will." In other words, it might be best for infertile women not to reproduce. I've actually heard several doctors speculate that infertility may be nature's way of preventing birth anomalies.

These sorts of comments disturb me for two reasons. First, this idea is unsupported by science.[1] There is no evidence to suggest that

---

[1] An excellent comparative review of birth anomalies associated with spontaneous pregnancy and IVF can be found in *IVF Children: The First Generation Assisted Reproduction and Child Development* by Alistair G. Sutcliffe (New York: The Parthenon Publishing Group, 2002).

assisted pregnancies have contributed to a significant increase in the incidence of birth anomalies in the general population, although relatively little research has been completed in this area.[2] As more and more ART children reach maturity, a more definitive assessment will be possible. In the meantime, fertility specialists around the world are helping to deliver beautiful, healthy babies. In waiting rooms everywhere, bulletin boards display scores of pictures of thriving infants who were born with the assistance of new technologies. Clearly, having a healthy baby is not only possible for many infertile couples; it is quite likely. Second, the suggestion that individuals shouldn't consider using ART is disturbing because women and men who are having difficulty conceiving or sustaining a pregnancy need medical professionals to be on their side, unequivocally, as committed as their patients are to overcoming their infertility.

The importance of emotional support for infertile patients should be obvious to physicians. Yet many doctors and clinics still don't offer their patients adequate psychological help. I believe that education, emotional preparation, and ongoing counseling for infertile patients might actually enhance the outcome of the ART process by reducing levels of stress hormones. Alice Domar, Ph.D., Director of the Mind/Body Center for Women's Health at Boston IVF has explored the effects of stress management on infertility in her excellent book, *Conquering Infertility*.[3] A positive mind body connection can work for patients not just on a psychological level, but by altering the body's chemistry at a cellular level, as well.

Infertile men and women need to take a proactive, independent role in finding appropriate guidance. I can't stress too much the importance of this. Having an open, comfortable, one-on-one

---

[2] There is a brief discussion of recent research findings on this subject, along with source citations, under the heading "The Unknowns with ART" at the end of this chapter.

[3] Alice D. Domar, Ph.D. and Alice Lesch Kelly, *Conquering Infertility: Dr. Alice Domar's Mind/Body Guide to Enhancing Fertility and Coping with Infertility* (New York: Viking Books, 2000).

relationship with a trusted confidante can make all the difference, not only in how you weather the journey to parenthood, but also in your overall, long-term psychological health. Make no mistake, infertility leaves a mark. Sooner or later, deep-seated emotional issues will surface. If you're considering using donated eggs or sperm, for example, you may need to mourn the loss of your ability to pass on your genetic heritage. Or you may need to overcome an old assumption that infertility is God's will before you can accept that you have a right to do something about it.

Of course, the most important source of emotional support for a woman struggling with infertility is her husband or partner. It is essential that her husband or partner be fully involved and wholeheartedly supportive. This involvement and support may not be present from the first moment that issues of infertility arise, nor from the first moment that the use of ART is considered, but for most loving couples it builds with time and with good communication. Without the eventual involvement and support of a husband or partner, overcoming infertility through ART will be extremely difficult, if not impossible. The full support of a husband or partner is seldom enough, however. Even the closest couples will find that they need the emotional support from third parties.

Where should you look for this support? There is no "right" answer to this question. You may discover the empathetic listener you need in a therapist, a member of the clergy, a good friend or understanding family member, or perhaps in a member of an infertility support group such as RESOLVE, accessible via the Internet. With each of these alternatives, there are many factors to consider.

Professionals. You may need to interview several counselors before you find one that's a good fit. You should ask whether the counselor has had training and experience in reproductive medicine. The American Society for Reproductive Medicine (ASRM), web site: www.asrm.org/Patients/topics/counseling.html provides a list of mental health professionals who offer infertility counseling. Counselors with this training will be familiar with the risks and benefits of procedures you may be offered, and they will anticipate and understand the emotional difficulties that may arise. A counselor with the appropriate training will be able to help you to make better, more informed decisions about your care. For example, an important decision you might face is whether to undergo the risk of selective embryo reduction. Your counselor should be familiar with the risks of higher order pregnancies (twins, triplets, etc.), as well as the risks of selective reduction procedures. He or she should be able to discuss the pros and cons of each option with you. If you are hesitant to accept these risks, or if you have difficulty with the idea of selective reduction, then you may want to tell your doctor that you don't want to transfer more embryos than you can safely carry.

Another area to investigate should you need third party assistance is what views the mental health counselor may have regarding selection of anonymous vs. known donor. Parents need to be able to sort through the pros and cons of both options without having to factor counselor bias into their thinking. At the time that I was seeking advice regarding ovum donation, there was a clear bias in favor of using an anonymous donor. Today, this bias appears to be less prevalent.

Another critical area to examine is the counselor's opinion about the advisability of parental disclosure of conception history to children of ART, and more importantly, what language to use in speaking with ART children about their origins. This is another area where the "conventional wisdom" is still evolving. In the 1950s, when sperm insemination first became available, nearly all doctors advised against disclosing to a child that he or she had been conceived with the help of a sperm donor. This advice was based both on the belief that a child conceived via sperm donation would be unlikely to uncover that fact, as well as the assumption that concealing this history would somehow help the child bond with his or her parents and prevent the development of identity confusion. By the time this first generation of children grew up, however, this assumption began to change, largely due to lessons learned in the adoption arena.

For several decades now, disclosure to adopted children about the circumstances of their birth and adoption has been regarded as appropriate and wise. More recently, with the advent of open adoption, disclosure to adopted children of the identities of their birth parents has also become common and accepted. It is probably safe to say that, in the adoption arena, full disclosure of all available information is rapidly becoming the psychological gold standard.

The issues surrounding disclosure, however, are not exactly the same for ART parents as they are for the parents of adopted children. These differences are discussed in Chapter 4. When selecting a counselor, ART parents should be aware that some therapists with an adoption counseling background, and with little experience in ART counseling, may not understand these differences and may therefore offer advice that is not always appropriate.

Web sites. When I was confronted with the emotional fallout from my donor-assisted pregnancy, I found it especially helpful to communicate with others who had shared a similar experience. There are web sites, like that of RESOLVE at www.resolve.org, or TASC (The American Surrogacy Center) at www.surrogacy.com, that can put you in touch with women who have been down every path of the journey through infertility. But remember, although these women may provide a wealth of practical information, they can't offer professional advice. Beware also of chat room contributors or web sites offering nutritional supplements or programs of exercise and meditation that promise to "cure" your infertility or help you get pregnant.

Relatives and friends. If you decide to seek advice and support from a relative or friend, choose someone who has already proven to be an excellent listener with a wise and thoughtful perspective. When you're feeling raw and vulnerable, it is not the time to experiment. Make your needs and expectations clear at the outset. If all you need is an opportunity to vent from time to time and you aren't looking for advice, be sure the confidant you've chosen understands this. Above all, be sure to make absolutely clear, from the beginning, your need for confidentiality, and always select someone whom you can trust to keep confidences.

Physicians, clergy, licensed therapists and counselors are required by the ethics of their professions to keep whatever you choose to share with them confidential. This is not true of friends and relatives. Even if confidentiality does not seem especially important to you as you begin your journey through infertility, you should recognize that your feelings on this subject might change as you struggle with choices along the way. It is always best to insist on confidentiality from others so that the decisions relating to what, when, and how to disclose are always yours to make.

In a recent Yale University Medical School study of parents by oocyte (egg) donation, it was found that significantly more women than men told others about using a donor to conceive, but two thirds of both the women and the men reported that they would not tell others if they had to do it over again.[4]

This subject receives a great deal of comment from women who participate in chat room discussions. As one woman put it, "Once the cat is out of the bag, you can't put it back in."

I love this poem from an anonymous author about a mother's yearning to have another baby.

Just Once More

I'd like to be pregnant just once more.
I'd like to see a plus sign on a pregnancy test and do a dance of joy on the bathroom floor.
I'd like to tell my husband, "We did it," and see the joy on his face.

---

[4] S.C. Klock and D.A. Greenfield, 'Parents' Knowledge About the Donors and their Attitudes Toward Disclosure in Oocyte Donation," *Human Reproduction*, July 2004, 19(7): 1575-1579.

I'd like to walk with my secret in those early months, a proud grin on my face, inexplicable to those who do not know.

Just once more, I would like to be more animal than human, connected to all living mothers in fur or in skin.

Just once more, I'd like to fold tiny clothes, change tiny diapers.

I'd like to help my daughter hold this new baby for the first time.

I'd like to see my husband sway an infant in his massive arms.

I'd like to fill the house with baby things: blankets and toys, a swing and a bassinet.

I'd like to feel the relief of getting a child to sleep, finally, and the tension of checking for breath throughout the night.

Just once more, I'd like to host the visitors, the well wishers, the gift bringers.

I'd like to hold my newest child up proudly for viewing.

I'd like to see my mother cry at the miracle of this new life.

I'd like to hand the baby to my husband so that I could hold and cradle my daughter.

I'd like to tell her about the time she was as small and needy as her new sibling, and how we tended her as gently.

Just once more, I'd like to let love multiply.

Identifying Infertility

Infertility is not usually the result of a single condition to be diagnosed, sorted out, and treated in a few office visits. Often during an evaluation, contributing factors are discovered for both male and female. And, as we age, our bodies can develop new conditions requiring that the original treatment plan be redirected. For example, sometimes a patient will have gone through a battery of diagnostic tests that find nothing definitive to explain her infertility, yet she remains unable to conceive. Then, we discover, perhaps two or three years down the road on a repeat uterine ultrasound in preparation for embryo transfer, that her uterine lining now needs additional hormonal support to allow a pregnancy to implant. Sometimes we discover that a patient has developed an immune component to her infertility, and although she can now conceive, she repeatedly miscarries. At other times, we find that the male partner has developed a significant infertility factor that requires us to use ICSI (intracytoplasmic sperm injection), a fertilization technique that introduces a single sperm into the oocyte. (For those who wish to read in more detail about the basic facts of infertility, including a description of common tests and procedures, see Appendices I and II.)

Who are the Infertile?

In some instances, patients have known from the time they were young that they would be unable to conceive due to a congenital problem. Others might learn of their infertility as a new condition subsequent to an illness or an operation that impacts their ability to either carry or conceive a child. And then there is the growing group of older female patients who find that their biologic clocks have been ticking much faster than they had imagined. They discover they will require specialized fertility assistance to achieve a successful pregnancy. In recent years, single women and gay and lesbian couples have also joined the ranks of the infertile seeking assisted conception or gestation in order to build families. Although they may not have suffered the same kinds of trauma associated with long standing infertility, nevertheless they bring to the table their own unique issues in seeking to start families and raise emotionally healthy children.

When to Seek Help Getting Pregnant

If a woman has been entirely healthy, with regular menstrual cycles, and has been timing intercourse carefully[5] to coordinate with ovulation, yet still cannot conceive, I recommend that she consult with a doctor after one year if she's younger than 35, and after six months if she's 35 years or older.

All the media stories about celebrity moms who miraculously have babies late in life have given many women a false sense of hope and security. The impression created—that if a woman is healthy and fit at 40, with a youthful body, her eggs will be fit and youthful too—just isn't so. By age 36 to 40, a woman's remaining supply of ova is rapidly losing the ability to be properly fertilized. A healthy lifestyle isn't going to affect whether or not an egg divides into the normal complement of chromosomes during final egg maturation and after fertilization.

In younger women, 20-25% of embryos conceived are chromosomally defective. They either fail to implant or go on to be miscarried. In women over 40, the incidence of chromosomal anomalies rises to 50-80%. The message is clear: Biology rules. A woman's egg cells are on their own time clock.

Who's your Doctor? Ob/Gyn vs. Specialist

You'll need to decide early on who will treat your infertility problem, an obstetrician/gynecologist (Ob/Gyn) or a fertility specialist known as a reproductive endocrinology and infertility (REI) specialist. Critical time and chances of conceiving can be lost for some women who linger too long with an Ob/Gyn before turning to an REI specialist. Just as a patient with a confirmed diagnosis of cancer should seek the care of an oncologist, a woman who is racing

---

[5] Intercourse should be timed every other day between days 10 and 18 of a normal 28-day cycle.

her biological clock and near the end of her reproductive years, or a couple facing certain confirmed infertility conditions, would be better off in the hands of a board certified, reproductive endocrinology and infertility specialist.

Are You Ready for ART?

This can be a tricky question. When has the right moment arrived to take the creation of your child's life out of the darkness of the womb and into the light of the lab? I believe it's whenever a woman:

- has had normal test results, is over age 35, and is unable to conceive after three to four attempts with intrauterine insemination and an ovulation inducing medication;
- has had three or more consecutive miscarriages without a clear diagnosis (e.g., due to incompetent cervix, genetic problem with fetus, etc.);
- fails to conceive within a year of treatment for known pathology up to age 35; or
- fails to conceive within six months of treatment for known pathology over age 35

Some couples turn to adoption at this point. Others elect to try ART. ART comes in many forms, can be very expensive, and comes with no guarantee of success. And success through ART can mean a number of different things depending on the reasons for a couple's infertility, the procedures selected, and the outcomes that are acceptable to the couple.

Most ART procedures involve in vitro fertilization (IVF). IVF includes all procedures that involve the retrieval of eggs from a woman and sperm from a man and the fertilization of egg by sperm in a Petri dish in the laboratory. ICSI (intracytoplasmic sperm injection) is a form of IVF. ZIFT (zygote intrafallopian transfer) is also a form of IVF because the zygote is the fertilized egg before it cleaves and becomes an embryo. GIFT (gamete intrafallopian transfer), on the other hand, does not involve IVF because the gametes, which are the egg and the sperm, are transferred to the fallopian tube before fertilization. Since fertilization will occur in the fallopian tube with GIFT, this form of ART is popular among those with religious beliefs mandating "natural conception." In general, because of increasing success rates of IVF with embryo transfer (ET), procedures such as GIFT and ZIFT are slowly becoming obsolete.

For most couples, ART starts with IVF, which involves nurturing the development of fertilized eggs, sometimes called oocytes or ova, to embryo stage in the laboratory, and then transfer of embryos into the uterus of the woman who will carry and deliver the child. To proceed with IVF, you need healthy eggs in sufficient quantity so that after fertilization there are a good number of embryos for transfer. The number of good embryos for transfer will depend on the donor's age. Your REI specialist may also try for additional embryos so that some can be frozen for future transfers if the initial transfer attempt fails.

Usually, the process of in vitro fertilization begins with drugs that will suppress natural hormonal cycling so that the ovaries can be stimulated with other drugs to produce many eggs in a single cycle. Suppression of the hormonal cycle, preparation of the uterus, and stimulation of the ovaries are usually accomplished through a combination of oral medications, and subcutaneous and/or intramuscular injections in the thighs, buttocks, or abdomen. In cases of donated eggs or embryos, the recipient's medications will not involve ovarian stimulation but will be just for the purpose of preparing the uterus for embryo transfer and implantation. All of these medications can be self administered at home. However, some of the injections can cause some discomfort and bruising, particularly when progesterone in oil or heparin is used. Thus, some women elect to have them administered by a nurse in an office or clinic setting.

The actual procedure for harvesting eggs can be carried out in an outpatient setting under light sedation and local anesthesia. The ovaries are first located using an ultrasound probe that is inserted towards the back of the vagina. A hollow needle is extended from the tip of the probe through the back wall of the vagina to reach each ovary. The follicles are then aspirated (emptied by suction), and as many eggs as possible are retrieved. These are immediately transferred to the laboratory where they are counted and assessed prior to fertilization.

The actual meeting of ovum and sperm occurs in a Petri dish after the sperm have been properly prepared. The fertilization of the ovum is usually facilitated by an embryologist, a key member of the REI specialist's team. In recent years, embryologists have become so proficient that fertilization can be accomplished with activation and injection of a single sperm directly into an ovum. This is done using a micropipette under microscopic guidance and is called intracytoplasmic sperm injection or ICSI.

Finally, the REI specialist will transfer the embryos into the mother's womb (or, if a gestational carrier is to be used, into the womb of the carrier) on the third, fifth, or sixth day following fertilization. (See Chapter 5 for a discussion of both gestational carriers and surrogates.) Then, in many cases an interminable two weeks must pass before it can be known if the procedure was successful.[6] Once a viable pregnancy is achieved, the mother-to-be (or gestational carrier) can return to her regular Ob/Gyn for prenatal care.

Unfortunately, not all IVF procedures work, and a couple's hopes may be raised by early promising signs, only to be dashed. After a promising egg retrieval and transfer of healthy embryos, the level of human chorionic gonadotropin (hCG), a hormone produced by the cells of the placenta as it develops, begins to rise. This rise is monitored by simple blood tests. Some women will experience a rise in hCG indicating a pregnancy, but the levels don't continue climbing at the predicted rate. This could be a sign of impending miscarriage, or it might signal a pregnancy that has implanted in the fallopian tube. Multiple ultrasounds and further blood tests will be performed to help determine what is happening with the pregnancy.

---

[6] Sometimes blood tests can confirm a pregnancy as early as eleven days.

If the hCG levels rise at a higher rate than expected, a woman may discover at the time of her ultrasound that there is more than one viable pregnancy. Over the next few weeks, she may be in limbo, waiting to find out just how many fetuses will continue growing. Often with multiple pregnancies, some of the gestational sacs will disappear. This can be a quiet process of embryo resorption into the mother's body, or it can present as a miscarriage accompanied by considerable bleeding.

Since the birth of my son via ovum donation in 1996, I have become a regular visitor to several of the confidential support groups on the Internet restricted to women who are struggling with problems of infertility or who have had children through ART. In one of my visits, I found this compelling story:

> *"I was just five weeks post transfer of four embryos and due for my ultrasound the next day, when I went to return some library books and felt a sudden warm gush while waiting at the check out counter. I knew I was bleeding. I raced home, called my husband, and put myself to bed. If the bleeding meant that I was miscarrying, I didn't want to lose all my healthy embryos.*
>
> *As we made our way to our scheduled ultrasound the next day, I kept praying that at least one little guy would have held on. I told my unborn children how sorry I was that some or even all of them might have had to let go. I thanked each one in my mind for trying his or her best.*
>
> *With the ultrasound, two tiny heartbeats were found. My husband and I were cautiously joyful. My bleeding eventually subsided as the pregnancy progressed. There are times, even today, when I look at our dear little boys, that I think about their two little brothers or sisters who didn't survive. I wonder what they would have looked like and imagine how close they would have felt to one another."*

Not everyone is so lucky. Sometimes uterine bleeding is accompanied by persistent cramping, and some or all the embryos can be dislodged. Usually miscarriage of "bad embryos" is nature's way of taking care of something that isn't normal. At other times, uterine bleeding may be a sign that a pregnancy is ectopic, located outside the uterus. Even healthy embryos cannot be saved if they implant in the fallopian tube. If a tubal pregnancy is discovered early enough, it can sometimes be dissolved by medication alone. If not, then the pregnancy must be carefully removed surgically so as to spare as much damage to the tube as possible. In some cases, the tube has been so extensively damaged that it has to be removed as well. Some doctors prefer this treatment, because it can prevent the risk of a repeated pregnancy in the affected tube.

For some women, the experience of getting as far as a **chemical pregnancy** (a rise in hCG without visual confirmation of pregnancy by ultrasound) or even a **clinical pregnancy** (a rise in hCG and confirmation by ultrasound of a gestational sac or developing embryo) is somehow encouraging, even if the pregnancy fails to progress. They feel that the early rise in hCG is a success and a sign that they should keep on trying. For others, the eventual drop in hCG and subsequent resorption of the embryo or miscarriage is crushing, almost too agonizing to bear.

If you achieve an early pregnancy through IVF only to lose the pregnancy, your physician can help you understand what went wrong and what the underlying causes may have been. He/she can give you information you will need in weighing the decision to try again. But only you can make this decision, and only you can decide if you have the emotional reserves to continue on a journey for which no outcome can be guaranteed.

The Unknowns with ART

Medical problems or conditions caused by the intervention of a physician are known as iatrogenic problems or conditions. Is it possible that procedures used to facilitate pregnancy through ART could result in iatrogenic conditions in ART children? Yes, it's possible.

For some ART procedures that have been in use for decades, there are ample reassuring data that suggest that the procedures are safe. For more recent procedures, the data are less complete.

Medicine is both art and science, and it evolves slowly through trial and error. Fortunately, the serious "errors" are relatively rare, but they do occur. A classic example in my specialty is the use of diethylstilbestrol (DES) in the 1940s, 50s, and 60s to prevent miscarriages in women with a history of prior miscarriages. More than 4.8 million women took DES prescribed by their physicians who believed that the drug was safe and would help their patients retain a viable pregnancy and deliver a healthy baby. Years later, it was discovered that the adult daughters of women who took DES had structural cervical abnormalities making it difficult for them to have successful pregnancies themselves. They were also found to be at significant risk for developing a particular kind of reproductive tract cancer called clear cell adenocarcinoma of the cervix and/or vagina. Because these problems did not surface until the children of DES moms reached adulthood, early identification of the problems through research was not possible.

There is some early evidence to suggest that IVF procedures are associated with an increased incidence of certain rare congenital anomalies in the general population.[7] But the overall increase in numbers of infants born with such anomalies is quite small because the initial incidence of the anomaly is quite rare. Nevertheless, anyone choosing ART should understand and accept that there are unknowns about the long-term results of the newer ART procedures.

Some of us make important decisions by engaging in a sort of cost-benefit analysis. The benefits of ART are easy to describe: the joy and fulfillment that will come with the birth of the child for whom we have been longing. It is the costs part that is more difficult. I think of these costs as having three components. The first is the financial component. These costs are reasonably predictable. The second is

---

[7] A growing body of research suggests some causal relationship between IVF procedures and certain congenital abnormalities. For an over view of the research to date, see: http://www.i-sis.org.uk/wwwART.php.

the emotional component. These costs are less predictable and can be enormous if success comes only after multiple attempts. The last part is the cost of risks, known or unknown, being realized. These risks include the known risk of failure to become pregnant and deliver a healthy baby and the still unknown risk that unpredicted problems will present themselves years later when the baby is an adult.

When my husband and I were making the decision to turn to ART, we didn't consciously engage in a cost-benefit analysis, but we did think about the emotional costs associated with failure, and we did think about the risks associated with new procedures.

Because of my professional training, I knew that my donor's egg would undergo some manipulation during the process of retrieval and evaluation and also at the time of assisted hatching. I knew that ZIFT (zygote intrafallopian transfer) involves the use of a different growth medium in the laboratory than that used for GIFT (gamete intrafallopian transfer). I also knew that ICSI (intracytoplasmic sperm injection) involves activating the sperm and then injecting it forcefully through the ovum wall with a needle after application of a special enzyme to the ovum wall. These and other procedures expose sperm, egg, gamete, zygote, or embryo to chemical, mechanical, and environmental factors (epigenetic factors) that are different in a number of respects from the corresponding factors that characterize natural, in vivo, fertilization and early development. Might these factors influence the way certain genes interact, for example?[8]

ICSI, GIFT, ZIFT: ART now includes a virtual smorgasbord of scientific options, all designed to improve the chances for success. How do you choose what is right? For me, the decision was based on two simple principles. They are: 1) always use the simplest and most proven procedure that yields a reasonable chance at success given the nature of the infertility problem, and 2) always select procedures and treatment based solely on patient needs, bearing in mind that a clinic sometimes bases procedure recommendations, and even patient

---

[8] For a more detailed discussion of epigenetic factors, see: http://www.hopkinsmedicine.org/press/2002/November/epigenetics.htm.

selection, on its own preferences for certain new procedures or its interest in improving its outcome statistics.[9]

Here's how applying these principles worked for me. In my case there was no male factor infertility involved. My husband had fathered two living children with me in earlier years. He was now 49 and in the interim had had no serious medical illnesses. So for me, when ICSI was offered, I said no. There was no reason for it. When I was offered the option of a five-day blastocyst transfer with higher likelihood of successful implantation following transfer, I also said no. Although the miscarriage rate for three-day old embryo transfers was somewhat higher than that for five-day old blastocyst transfers, I preferred the option of my uterus doing mother nature's job of culling out the less fit embryos on her own. I wondered if there might be something about the laboratory environment during days four and five that would interfere with this natural selection process, or if the five-day embryos might be otherwise altered by their lives in the laboratory in ways that my body would be unable to recognize.

On the other hand, when I was offered assisted hatching,[10] I elected to have this particular procedure because my physician recommended it. I understood his recommendation to be based on the fact that my embryos were not top grade and his belief that assisted embryo hatching prior to transfer would improve the chances of a successful pregnancy and birth. When I made this decision back in 1995, I was 49, one of the oldest patients he had treated, so the procedure made sense for me.

---

[9] Some clinics specialize in certain types of treatment and therefore tend to recommend those treatments. Some clinics will not accept patients with a low chance of success, either because they do not specialize in the treatments best suited to those patients, or because they are trying to improve their statistics (e.g., live births per ART cycles started).

[10] Assisted hatching involves altering, by mechanical or chemical means, the outer shell of the embryo before transfer so that by the time it is placed back in the uterus the outer shell breaks open (hatches), allowing the embryo cells to burrow their way into the lining of the uterus.

I understood that science didn't have answers to all my questions, and I knew that some of my choices were based as much on feelings or instinct as on thoughtful analysis, but I felt comfortable with the way I made my decisions. Fortunately, my husband and I were blessed with a beautiful, healthy boy. Today he is ten, and he continues to thrive. If someday he should develop a disease or condition that is found to be linked to some aspect of ART, my husband and I will deal with that without recriminations or efforts to lay blame. I believe that we have approached the key medical decisions with care and love, and that belief will, I think, make it easier for us to live with whatever the future holds.[11]

YOU WILL FIND A WAY:
Tara's encouraging words

"You and your husband will find a path, no matter what. And any child who meets your arms will be blessed. Just think years forward about how amused and amazed your children will be to think of the struggles you underwent to become their very own special parents. Like all children, they will want to know their roots. But in the final analysis, they will know that what counts in life is that there are many ways to build a family, and they are where they are because they were wanted. Donors, gestational carriers, even those whose loving touches created a new life they could not care for, are all part of the miracle that helps your babies reach their mommy's and daddy's arms. That's the true story of the family of man."

---

[11] At the time of our son's delivery, we cryopreserved his cord blood so the stem cells contained in the cord blood would be available to him to treat any diseases or conditions he might develop in the future. New treatments using stem cells are continuously evolving. (We would have done this for our older children had the option been available when they were born.)

Chapter 2

When the Heart Calls: Battling Infertility

Facing the Emptiness: Dealing with Yourself

Celeste has been trying to become pregnant for more than two years. She's been through two surgeries to open her fallopian tubes and has undergone artificial insemination six times—all without success. But at age 33, she's not ready to give up on having a baby.

"I have a biological urge to procreate," she writes on the bulletin board in the chat room of her online infertility support group. "I yearn for the mystical experience of feeling a flutter beneath my ribs, hearing the sound of my baby's heartbeat, and one day seeing the face of my child. The thought of not having children leaves me feeling cold and empty, without hope. What is the point of life if not to share it with children?"

Celeste expresses the deep, instinctual, universal desire to be a parent. When infertility enters the picture, this unfulfilled longing can become excruciating. In fact, the inability to conceive presents such tremendous challenges that mental health professionals consider it a major life crisis, as traumatic as dealing with the death of a loved one or a life-threatening illness. The emotional highs and lows are like a roller coaster—except there's nothing fun about them. In the early stages of the quest for a baby, there may be lots of options; then time passes, and with each failure, hope diminishes. Grief and pain intensify, and the desire to have the parenting experience can become an overwhelming, all-consuming one.

Celeste continues. "I've found myself in dark moments wondering if God isn't really trying to tell me something. Maybe I'm not meant to be a mother. Maybe I would damage a child. Maybe I don't deserve a baby. Maybe I'm being punished for some unknown sin. Maybe I don't WANT a baby hard enough. Maybe I'm asking for too much. GOD, PLEASE, WHY CAN'T I JUST HAVE A HEALTHY BABY OF MY OWN?"

"What is wrong with me? What did I do to deserve this? Whatever it is, I'll fix it, I promise. I'll smile as I throw up, I won't complain through labor, and I'll NEVER, EVER criticize my darlings, and . . . . No, that is a bunch of hooey. I'm human. I'm not perfect. But no one else on the planet is, either. And a whole bunch of them have babies, and I don't. And that SUCKS."

"I know that infertility has been around forever. The Bible records a lot of women who suffered through it. History mentions a ton, too. I am NOT special because I am STERILE. So, why do I still experience those moments in time when I would bargain my soul for a BABY? Why do I still wonder if I DESERVE a child?"

For Celeste and others struggling with infertility, getting a handle on this kind of thinking—"Because I am sterile, I must not deserve a baby of my own."—can be difficult.

Infertility challenges a woman's identity, self-image, and sense of self-worth. Many women go through childhood and adolescence with happy images of adult years filled with the laughter of children and the joy of being a mother. This is very often true, as well, for those women who choose to pursue a demanding profession or career. They frequently think in terms of when to start a family, not if they should have children. The role of loving mother is every bit as important for them as is the role of competent professional in shaping the self-image that is a constant in their lives and that contributes to their emotional stability and security. And the emotional challenge that comes with a woman's realization that she is infertile is often compounded by the typically painful, invasive infertility procedures and treatments, some of which will alter her hormonal balance, leaving her depressed and emotionally labile.

Infertility can be equally difficult for men. When the problem lies with the woman, her spouse is often left feeling powerless and isolated, relegated to the role of helpless onlooker. When the problem is male infertility, the emotional challenges to the man are different. For those men who see themselves as heads of their families and protectors of their spouses, infertility raises questions about their place in the world and their manhood. It is often experienced as weakness and inadequacy.

As a general rule, men have a harder time than women dealing with the emotions that are stirred up by infertility. Not all men suffer in silence, however. When Robert learned that his wife, Patti, a cancer survivor, would never be able to conceive or carry a pregnancy, he acknowledged his grief to an online support group. "I always imagined seeing in my child some of the wonderful genes my wife might have passed on, but now I must let go of that for both of us. It's not just about genes. I feel for my wife, who will never know the experience of bearing a child we created together. Birth represents one of the primal, shared passages that we will deeply miss."

Just by expressing himself, Robert is doing important emotional work. This sort of painful emotional work is critically important for both women and men. Allowing yourself to confront difficult feelings and accept them as part and parcel of the journey will enable you to keep moving forward. That, in turn, will help guide you to the resolution that's right for you, whether it's a pregnancy achieved through ART, a family created through adoption, or a decision to live childfree.

Fielding Feedback: Dealing with Outsiders

A big question for couples with a fertility problem is whom to tell, and how much. Be prepared to discover, if you haven't already, that revealing your infertility means exposing yourself to foolish and hurtful remarks. Family members, friends, and colleagues may intend to be helpful, but their advice and comments are often based on myths, misconceptions, and ignorance. Or their attitudes may reflect their own discomfort about your situation. I've found that the best defense is to have an answer rehearsed and ready for the obvious questions. You'll also need to learn how to ignore and forgive hurtful remarks.

All the same, it's infuriating to hear comments like "Just relax, it will happen," when you've endured so much to become pregnant and you know so well that infertility is a disease of the reproductive system, not a nervous condition. And the comment "You want kids? Take one of mine," which is meant to be funny, is seldom amusing to someone still longing for children.

Women trying to become pregnant in their mid to late 40s, when their eggs may no longer be viable, are likely to face either overt or implied criticism over the timing of their efforts to have children. Annette, who became a mother at age 50 when many of her friends were becoming grandmothers, describes her experience in an Internet chat room: "Many of your friends your age will think you've lost your marbles if you start speaking about trying to build a family. They're likely to say, 'Let it alone, it's pushing the envelope.' Or they'll give you a look that says, 'Is it really appropriate at your age?'" She offers this advice to women like her: "You've got to accept that there's not the same level of peer support out there for you now as there would have been had the current technological options been available when you were younger and struggling with your infertility. But take heart, it's not all bad. You've lived enough of life to know that you don't have all the answers, and you've probably developed enough of a sense of humor and grace to know when to be tenacious, when to roll with the punches, and how to adapt to unforeseen circumstances. Good qualities for upcoming parenthood!"

One of the most frequently heard questions is: "Why don't you adopt? There are lots of deserving children who need homes." This is a question everyone who's infertile is likely to hear sooner or later. Marion, a mom-by-adoption and an adoption counselor who holds seminars for prospective adoptive parents, has developed a pointed response. To anyone who asks an infertile individual, "Why don't you adopt?" she quickly shoots back, "Why don't you? You seem to have a wonderful family; a child would be lucky to join you." She says it sweetly, with a smile, but she means for it to sting. She dislikes the assumption that because a woman is having trouble conceiving, she should be responsible for the global issues of homeless children and an overcrowded planet.

I agree. No one should be made to feel guilty because of a medical condition. Infertile couples have the right to choose how they will build their families. And, as with any couple, their choice is a personal and private decision.

In any case, for many infertile couples, adoption is not an either/or proposition. They pursue adoption as they seek to conceive through ART; they're committed to becoming a parent any way they can.

Allegra is one of the women with whom I have been corresponding via e-mail. She's been battling infertility for many years and has several signs hanging near her desk to help her remember how to respond to negative feedback. They read:

"Don't tell me what I want or how I should feel."

"It's my timing, it's my life, it's my family."

"In the midst of the trials and despair of this journey, only kindness and goodness are welcome."

"I am strengthening my resolve and smiling at my destiny."

I'd add one more: "This is my life and I'm in charge of my choices, no matter what anyone else has to say."

Keeping the Dream Alive

Just keeping up your spirits, in the face of invasive medical procedures and an insensitive world, can be a daunting task. Many of the couples I've talked to find a way to do this, using their imagination. Fran and her husband, for example, are pursuing a Chinese adoption at the same time they try to create a new life with the help of donated sperm and ova. One of the ways Fran copes is by imagining her future children.

"I dream about them off in the distance," she says. "My fantasies help me get ready for them. Someday, I'm sure I'll meet them. And I know they'll surprise me in ways I can't imagine. But until then, I dream. My mother, bless her, is helping too. We're months away from even having a photo of our Chinese child, but I imagine a daughter whom we'll name Kaleigh Marie. My dream baby received a onesie from Grandma a few weeks ago. It's bright pink, embroidered with little bunnies. It's beautiful and I can see my little girl wearing it someday."

Joyce, a gardener, tells me over coffee about a dream she had one night. "I was at the checkout counter in the grocery store, and the cashier scanned a packet of seeds. I looked at the brightly colored flowers on the package and saw that it was labeled 'Babies.' I woke up startled, realizing that was exactly what I'm doing. First, I'm getting my uterus ready, like rich, dark soil. When it's just right, I plant the seeds. And like the seeds in a real flower garden, there are no guarantees. Some seeds produce beautiful plants, some don't. I understand that, but there are always lots of expectations. I have to continue to wait and watch through the entire growing time, never giving up hope."

Joyce's dream reminds me of my own experience when I was trying to have my third child. At the time of embryo transfer, while I was lying on my back in the doctor's office and just letting my mind wander, I had a vision of our backyard garden in Hawaii, by the sea, with its rich, warm soil. As soon as the transfer was complete and I could go home, I went straight to that plot of earth. For the next two weeks, as I waited to hear whether or not the embryos had "taken" and I was pregnant, I tended it as never before. This intuitive, spiritual connection to Mother Earth was comforting to me and gave me a meaningful way to channel my dreams and desires.

Riding the Emotional Roller Coaster:
How to Support your Partner

The drive to have a child is a potent one—and it comes not only with an array of powerful feelings, but also with conflicting ones. Not surprisingly, a woman and her partner may sometimes find themselves at odds with each other. When Shelley and Ken arrived in my office for an initial consultation, they'd been under the care of another gynecologist for two years. Shelley, 44, had only occasional, irregular ovulation, and she'd been treated with a number of courses of a fertility drug to stimulate her ovaries, each time without success.

Time was precious for this couple. They both had been married previously, and each had children from the first union, but they wanted to have a baby together. Shelley was nearing the end of her ability to become pregnant with her own eggs. Her eggs were rapidly declining.

"I hate this running-out-of-time syndrome," she told me. "I find myself saying to Ken, 'Yes, let's give it one more try,' and then two days later telling him, 'No, let's give up and get on with our lives.' Mixed in there is the guilt I have about how much it's costing and that we should be spending the money on the children we already have. Ken, meanwhile, isn't ready to give up yet. He gets annoyed with me when I flip-flop. The days when we're at odds can feel very lonely."

"Don't misunderstand me," Shelley went on. "Ken and I love each other. Our other children aren't lacking for anything. But still, I feel with each of those negative cycles that we've spent time, energy, and money on a dream that can't come true. Ken doesn't agree with me at all. He thinks we're spending money on something we desperately want and that's all we need to consider."

With the help of a counselor, Ken and Shelley were able to move through her ambivalence and his frustration about her waffling. Eventually, Shelley came to treasure Ken's steadfast grasp on their dream. He, in turn, was encouraged to consider some of her more practical concerns.

In talking with infertile couples, I've noticed that frequently one partner focuses on the practical concerns while the other holds the vision. Teamwork like this is important, because each partner will have multiple decisions to make, and with all the challenges to face, they don't need to be at each other's throats. As Shelley and Ken talked through their thoughts and concerns, with a little guidance and support from their counselor, they did become a tight team. In the end, after careful consideration of all the factors—practical, medical, spiritual—they decided to seek the help of an REI (reproductive endocrinology and infertility) specialist and pursue an ovum donor assisted pregnancy. Fourteen months after that initial visit with me, Shelley gave birth to a six-pound baby girl.

In trying to help my patients cope with conflicting emotions surrounding the decision to pursue ART, I have found that emotions triggered by financial issues are often among the most difficult. There is, of course, the practical challenge of finding the many thousands of dollars that will likely be required to pay for the treatments and procedures. But, the angst associated with the necessary juggling of family finances is enormous for many couples; it can destabilize a marriage. Why is this?

All marriage or partnership relationships achieve stability through an allocation of roles and responsibilities that are acceptable to, and comfortable for, both parties. Who does the shopping? Who cooks? Who decides where to go on the next vacation? All couples work out their answers to these and a thousand similar questions. To a large degree, the answers to these sorts of questions, taken as a whole, define relationships. Some answers are important to some couples, but are relatively unimportant to other couples. But for most couples, the answers to the key financial questions are extremely important in defining a sense of balance within the marriage relationship. These key financial questions are "Who earns the money to support the family?" and "Who decides how the family's money will be spent?" The answers to these questions are important because finances are the key to so many decisions that affect life style and social standing: where to live, what car to drive, what clubs to join. And the one who earns the money usually has the greater influence on how the money is spent and how these sorts of decisions are made.

This influence is often exerted subtly, hidden beneath a façade of apparent equality. With most couples, a comfortable equilibrium is reached where routine, day-to-day financial decisions are made jointly after open discussion and a weighing of pros and cons. But the decision to spend tens of thousands of dollars on ART is hardly a routine one, and the making of such a decision can upset a couple's equilibrium in ways that tend to bring to the surface any disparity in influence over financial matters.

In Ken and Shelley's marriage, it was Ken who was the money earner and the one with the most influence over financial decisions. He was also the one most committed to spending the family's savings in pursuit of the dream he shared with his wife. He was able to reassure Shelley that the expenditure was affordable and that she need not feel guilty about risking money that would otherwise have been saved for their other children.

It is somewhat more common to find a husband who is the primary earner and who is the one most reticent or cautious about investing in ART. This reticence or caution may be based on very real, practical concerns about family finances, but a wife who is desperate for a child may well experience this caution as an emotional abandonment or a blatant assertion of influence or power that upsets the family's normal equilibrium. One of my colleagues who counsels infertile couples reports that it is not uncommon for disagreements over the affordability of ART to escalate into marital discord that can lead to divorce. Needless to say, it is the emotional baggage that accompanies the making of difficult financial decisions that threatens relationships, not the financial issues themselves.

Reality Check: The Financial Costs

What are the costs of ART? Today, the average cost per cycle for stimulating ovaries with clomiphene citrate (CC), plus intrauterine insemination (IUI) is $500. The average cost per cycle with one of the drugs in the family of Human Menopausal Gonadotropin (hMG) plus IUI is $2,500. And the in vitro fertilization procedure (IVF), per cycle, can run from approximately $7,000 excluding medications to $13,000 or more with medications.

There are, of course, women who may be lucky enough to become pregnant after only a cycle or two of clomiphene citrate, but many women require many more tries, in addition to other complicated procedures. For these women, before a pregnancy is achieved, the tab can reach $50,000 or more. Even then, there are no guarantees for success.

Private adoption can cost anywhere from $2,000 to $30,000+ depending on how it is pursued. Many state adoptions are free but can involve toddlers or older children who have had one or more prior placements and who come with special needs.

A few insurance companies, depending on the state, may cover a wide range of infertility treatments, but most offer only limited help, especially with ART procedures. In some states, for example, couples with male infertility are excluded from treatment, as are single women. Although special interest groups are working to force broader coverage for infertility treatments, the insurance industry is resistant to change, and until this change occurs, for many couples the costs of IVF and other ART procedures will be prohibitive.

For these couples, the knowledge that ART is available but is financially out of reach is especially frustrating. "It's crazy-making," a friend's daughter told me. She was in tears because she had already reached the limits of what her husband's insurance would cover. "It's bad enough that I haven't been able to get pregnant after two years of trying," she said, both angry and heartbroken. "It seems doubly cruel that there's help out there that I can no longer access."

When I was trying to conceive via ovum donation in 1995, I considered several reproductive endocrinology and infertility clinics that reported good statistical success with women my age. I selected a clinic in San Francisco that had taken an innovative approach to marketing and had introduced, as an option, a qualified "money back guarantee" to patients that fell into a medically eligible candidate group. Because I had delivered healthy babies before, was in good health with no apparent uterine problems, was planning on ovum donation, and had a husband with no fertility issues, I was eligible for this new plan. For a fixed price of $16,000, excluding certain donor expenses, the clinic would perform the egg retrieval from my donor, the in vitro fertilization of the retrieved eggs with my husband's sperm, an initial fresh embryo transfer procedure, and three additional attempts (on successive cycles) to successfully implant any remaining embryos from the initial IVF procedure. If a successful pregnancy resulted from any of those attempts, the clinic would retain the full $16,000 fee. If a successful pregnancy did not result, approximately $11,000 would be refunded. The alternative, and the more normal practice, was a flat fee per attempt, with no refunds if all the attempts were unsuccessful.

The innovative, partial refund plan appealed to me, and I selected it. I was happy to pay $16,000 to become pregnant, and I knew I would not feel I had paid too much if I became pregnant on the first attempt. On the other hand, if I failed to become pregnant after four attempts, I would not feel that I had paid a significant sum with nothing to show for it. I was also reassured somewhat by the fact that the clinic I had chosen was willing to bet, in effect, on its ability to help me. (I became pregnant on the first cycle.)

In 1995, this "partial money back guarantee" plan was new and somewhat controversial. Today a number of clinics offer something similar, generally referred to as a "shared risk" plan. One clinic, for example, charges $13,400 for which the patient gets one "fresh cycle" and as many thawed embryo transfer cycles as necessary until the patient either gets pregnant or all the available frozen embryos are used up. If the patient does not become pregnant, refunds of up to 90% of the $13,400 fee are provided. The refund percentage varies according to the age of the donor.

Handling It Together

Couples who dream of parenthood and undertake ART will have to endure rigid schedules of injections, great expense, and often great disappointment. Some husbands are able to help their wives through the psychological and physical ordeal, some aren't. There's a lot of technical information to absorb, a multitude of decisions to make, a lot of waiting and uncertainty, and a great deal of emotional strain. It's easy to feel that life is spinning out of control under the stress, and it's common for a marriage to suffer.

ART is not a simple matter of going to the doctor once a week and then going home to wait for results. Many of the mechanical tasks of ART are done by the couples themselves. One of the biggest of these chores is injecting hormones—not a simple job. First of all, the woman has to follow a precise schedule that is likely to interfere with her normal workday. And injection sites can become painfully bruised over time. For some women, the process of sticking a needle into the thigh or abdominal wall with sufficient force is very difficult—and it may not be any easier for her partner.

Alana describes her experience: "I had to mark a large calendar with how much of which hormone to inject at what times on which days. I'd gotten the procedure itself down to a fine art by placing an icepack on my backside beforehand so the intended injection site would be sufficiently numbed. I even marked the intended target with an 'X' to help my husband's aim. But he would inevitably hesitate, fiercely staring at the 'X' before throwing the needle into me like a dart. By the time he had gotten up his nerve to strike the bull's eye, the numbness would be wearing off, and I'd have tightened my muscles reflexively, making it harder for the needle to get through. We finally gave up the team approach. I had to go it alone."

Most women require a combination of injections and vaginal suppositories to prepare the ovaries for egg retrieval and/or prepare the womb for implantation following embryo transfer. Sometimes, women are found to have auto-immune problems that place them at risk for rejecting a pregnancy. They may be advised to take additional medications such as aspirin (taken orally) or heparin (injected subcutaneously). It is important to note that clinics can differ in their philosophies about certain immunological treatments. Medications that address the immune system have benefits and risks that women should become familiar with in order to make a sound decision whether or not to use them.

Then there is the embryo transfer itself. Because this procedure is done under ultrasound guidance for careful visualization, the patient will be asked to have a full bladder beforehand. The doctor usually positions the woman on her back with her legs in stirrups. Although the transfer procedure usually isn't painful, some women may experience cramping, particularly if the doctor must place a clamp on the cervix to straighten out the canal leading into the uterus. A long, thin, flexible catheter is then guided through the cervix to the proper depth within the uterine cavity for embryo transfer. It is wonderful to have the presence of your partner at such a time. If you think you will feel anxious about the medical procedure, you can bring in a CD of your favorite relaxing music. Many women report that the moment of embryo placement carries with it deep emotions. Here's what I remember from my own experience:

Because my husband, David, and I needed to fly to San Francisco for our procedure, I wanted to make the emotional journey as wonderful as possible for us in all the little ways I could. The first step was to find a hotel in which I'd feel at home for the stay. I found something quaint, reasonably priced, and just quirky enough for my tastes, high up on Sacramento Street. It was a small hotel that had been around for ages, converted from two old elegant Victorian town-houses, containing bedrooms filled with unique baroque furnishings and private bathrooms with claw-foot tubs and heated towel racks. When I read that the stay would include fresh flowers in my room, nightly piano concerts, and a performing ghost, that clinched my choice.

During our transfer procedure, David and I played a CD we had chosen with some dolphin music. We watched in breathless wonder at the ultrasound screen as our embryos were gently coaxed out of the transfer tube into the safety of my womb. Mind you, we couldn't see the embryos—they were far too tiny for the naked eye—but it felt as if we could, and tears were flowing freely. The entire room seemed bathed in quiet reverence.

And Now the Wait

Next is the nearly two-week wait following transfer, a period during which every episode of cramping or spotting brings panic that a miscarriage is imminent. Women who felt nothing during the procedure and have no cramping or spotting afterwards still worry that their embryos won't implant, or that the embryos floating freely in the womb might somehow fall out or be pushed out. It's not unusual for a woman to be terrified of using the toilet following transfer, although, in reality, this is not a risk. Any pushing required to move the bowels will not cause expulsion of embryos from the uterus. The muscles used to void bowels or bladder do not significantly affect the uterus, and in any event, the cervix functions as an effective barrier, like a sealed door, between uterus and vagina.

Even if the embryo transfer procedure itself goes perfectly, the waiting period afterward feels interminable. Desperate for good news, and too eager to wait for the pregnancy test in the doctor's office, women perform one home pregnancy test after another, searching for that faint blue line. Repeated false negatives from these over-the-counter home test kits are quite common because the home test kits are insensitive compared to the blood tests performed in a doctor's office or clinic. Sometimes, in the early days after embryo transfer, a woman could also get a false positive test result because she had received an hCG injection. There is no getting around the wait.

Here is Nadia's description of the long wait:

"I am in the car. The mobile phone rings. It is my doctor. My heart literally feels as if it stops when he asks, 'Is this a good time to talk?' He proceeds to explain how the follicles are not growing much at all. 'Your ovaries are not acting like a typical 37-year-old's. We need to recheck your hormone levels.'

"'NO!' I want to scream. Though my brain is reeling, I gather my wits enough to pull over to the side of the road and grab a pen and write down the details that will lead me to my next decision, whether or not to cancel the cycle . . . .

"It is time for church, but I keep to myself; I look at no one, mostly because any human contact would make me cry right now. I pray that God might just make things clear to us. 'Just make your path known, God.'

"He does. By the time we return home, the message is there for us. The low hormone levels require that we cancel."

☼

"Another cycle has begun. This time we make it to transfer, but I am sure the pregnancy tests will be negative. What I don't realize is that hope dies hard, and although my mind is telling me my body isn't pregnant, my heart is hoping that I am. When the results come back 'less than one,' meaning not a chance of pregnancy, I break down. Once again, my world has crumbled, and pieces of me have crumbled as well.

"I suppose the pain of a negative pregnancy test is similar for all infertile couples. You ache with the unfairness of it all. I ask, 'What happened, God? Am I not special enough to warrant your help? Haven't we learned enough of your lessons?' Questions like this do not help and only serve to deepen the hurt. I tell my husband I would like to talk to our pastor, because I need some help before I give up on God altogether . . . .

"Well, as if this is not enough to fathom, I have now been told that the lab results were in error and we should restart our pregnancy support hormones at once! What is going on? Is this some kind of miracle?

"I am cautious. I wait for the follow-up tests to confirm the pregnancy. What a miracle of a rollercoaster! The lab test results are rising. Now, we wait for the ultrasound. It is more than five weeks along now, and we are about to see our baby's heart beating!

"The ultrasound shows life. A baby is growing, but it's in my fallopian tube! There is no way he can survive. He will be surgically taken away from me, removed, along with my tube. I have been given a taste of his life, and now I shall lose him . . . . This is by far the hardest blow yet."

It Takes Two

If a relationship is to survive, partners facing the challenges of ART need to think carefully, and keep an open mind, about how they're going to be there for each other. "If my husband weren't so dedicated to sharing every part of the experience with me," writes Sally, "it would be just too hard. He helps by doing little things, like leaving a glass of water on the nightstand for when I wake up thirsty in the night, or giving me an extra kiss or hug. And it goes both ways. I've found that the less stressed out I am, the less stressed out he is. So it's kind of a circle."

An online support mothers group makes the following suggestions for husbands and wives:

- Assume that you'll sometimes have misgivings, feel exhausted and hopeless. Those feelings are just part of the ART journey. It doesn't mean you're weak or reneging on your commitment to the process.
- Check in with each other from time to time and reflect on the process. Help each other be aware of how having a baby can become an obsession.
- Have fun with each other, and with friends and family—do things that have nothing to do with getting pregnant, things you used to do.
- Vent when you need to, but direct your anger towards the situation that has gone awry, not at each other. If you do find yourself taking out your frustrations on each other, find ways to forgive and move on.
- Know that you may not always agree about things along the way. Be each other's advocate anyway.
- Join an infertility support group together.
- Agree to seek counseling together if, in spite of these efforts, you are still feeling unsupported or unappreciated.

A Word about Intimacy

Couples should anticipate a change in their sex lives while the woman is undergoing treatment for infertility and during pregnancy if the treatment is successful. For many couples, the intense focus on infertility, and the accompanying preoccupation with the reproductive system and the mechanics and biology of procreation, are inconsistent with the spontaneity and playfulness of lovemaking. The result is a dampening of sexual ardor. This is quite common for women struggling with infertility, and many husbands find this difficult and frustrating.

Nor do issues relating to sexual activity abate once a clinical pregnancy is achieved. Many women have an almost irrational fear of dislodging a successfully implanted embryo or causing a miscarriage of a healthily growing fetus. As a result, they are less receptive to, and sometimes openly resist, their partners' sexual advances. This fear can be subconscious and can persist despite assurances from the woman's Ob/Gyn that gentle lovemaking after implantation is perfectly safe.

I recommend that couples undergoing treatment for infertility discuss the impact of such treatment on their sex lives both with their Ob/Gyn and with a counselor. Their Ob/Gyn can tell them when it is clinically advisable to refrain from sexual activity and when it is safe to have sex. A counselor can help them anticipate the strains on a relationship that typically occur when there is a change in frequency of sexual activity, and especially when there is a decrease in interest or receptivity on the part of either partner.

In counseling my patients who are having issues relating to sex, I have often called their husbands into my office and, after a frank discussion about the stresses caused by infertility, have pulled out a prescription pad and written a prescription for "home cooked candle light dinner, followed by cuddling AND NO SEXUAL INTERCOURSE, once per week." I tell them I will be checking with their wives to see if the prescription is being filled. Treating the issue with a touch of humor in this way tends to make it less threatening and to put it in perspective. And the romance-and-intimacy-without-intercourse prescription, if followed, often leads to a mutual discovery that there are ways to achieve love and intimacy, and even sexual gratification, that do not require sexual intercourse.

Another Happy Ending

Like Shelley and Ken and many other couples, Celeste, whom you met at the beginning of this chapter, and her husband worked with a specialist in infertility counseling to better manage the stress of her long-standing infertility. After her second IVF attempt, she became pregnant. The pregnancy was uncomplicated and, with the help of her Ob/Gyn, she delivered a healthy seven-pound boy. Celeste says now, "I'm sure I'd never have experienced the joy of my son's birth if it weren't for the help I received accepting my feelings about all those procedures and disappointments. Being able to visualize success lessened my stress and allowed my body to respond. It was an awakening of my mind/body connection—and a miracle."

The mind/body connection to which Celeste attributes her breakthrough with infertility is no fiction; this connection she describes is both real and powerful. Alice Domar, PhD, Director of the Mind/Body Center for Women's Health at Boston IVF and Assistant Professor in the Department of Obstetrics and Gynecology at Harvard Medical School, has extensively studied this relationship and the potential for improving fertility. In her book, *Conquering Infertility: Dr. Alice Domar's Mind/Body Guide to Enhancing Fertility and Coping with Infertility,* Dr. Domar describes the results of detailed studies exploring this connection and provides readers with the necessary tools to enhance this connection for themselves.

Chapter 3

The World of Assisted Reproductive Technology (ART)

What leaves you in awe? For me, it's the wonder of biology. How the sun nourishes life. How the moon, the tides, and the human body cycle in eternal rhythms. How a flower unfurls in delicate and perfect beauty. How a heartbeat sounds through a stethoscope, and how a living cell appears through a microscope. All of these things inspire reverence in me.

As an obstetrician, I am especially awed by reproduction. It is through reproduction that species are perpetuated and achieve a form of immortality. For most species, reproduction is instinctive, but for humans it is both instinctive and intentional. And when reproduction is intentional, it is one of the purest expressions of love. The love expressed through reproduction is not just the love that we feel for another person, it is the more substantial love that we demonstrate through sacrifice and commitment. In his book, *A Road Less Traveled,* psychiatrist M. Scott Peck defines love as "the will to extend one's self for the purpose of nurturing one's own or another's spiritual growth."[12]

---

[12] M. Scott Peck, *The Road Less Traveled* (New York: Simon & Schuster, 1978) 81.

I like this definition because it recognizes that love is both purposeful and reverent. This is the love that is expressed when a couple plans for, prepares for, and commits to the raising of a child.

Until recently, this very special expression of love was denied to a great many infertile couples. But over the past four to five decades, the development of assisted reproductive technology has made it possible for many such couples to realize their dreams and become parents. To my mind, this is science at its best—something wondrous and awe inspiring.

The Birth Matrix Chart on the following pages shows the various ways that it is now possible to conceive a child and start a family.

As you can see, it can take from two to five contributors to bring a baby to life. For fertile couples, it takes two, and for infertile couples whose need for ART is limited to medication or IVF, it also takes two. For infertile couples who need more extensive help, it can take as many as five. For these couples to become parents, the help and expertise of a number of other individuals will also be required: the REI specialist, the embryologist, the clinic staff, etc. Yet it's important to remember that for all ART babies, there is a hierarchy of responsibility, and a driving purpose behind the creation of a new life, that starts with the parents. And when that new life emerges, the ultimate responsibility belongs to the parents, and remains theirs exclusively.

Let me say it another way: It is my firm belief that regardless of how many contributors, or collaborators, or donors, or medical professionals may be involved in the conception and delivery of a child, every child has two parents—and only two.[13]

A baby brought to life through reproductive assisted technology exists only because of his or her parents' dedicated yearning to procreate. If it were not for the infertility that caused these parents to seek an alternative way to bring a child into their lives, their particular baby would never have been born. Donors and carriers are generous

---

[13] In the case of single mothers, the role of a donor or gestational carrier could be redefined as that of a "parent" if an ongoing family relationship is intended.

The Birth Matrix: An Illustrated Guide to All the Options

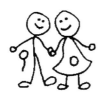

Spontaneous pregnancy

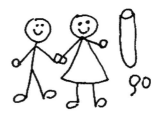

In vitro assisted pregnancy

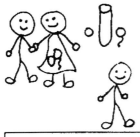

Donor sperm assisted pregnancy

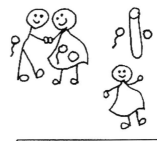

Donor ovum assisted pregnancy

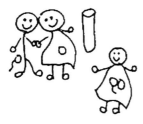

Gestational carrier assisted pregnancy

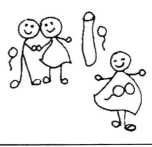

Traditional surrogate assisted pregnancy

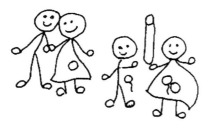

Donor sperm, gestational carrier assisted pregnancy

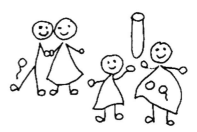

Donor ovum, gestational carrier assisted pregnancy

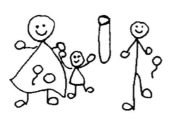

Single mother, donor sperm assisted pregnancy

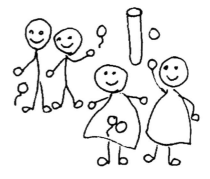

Gay male couple, gestational carrier assisted pregnancy

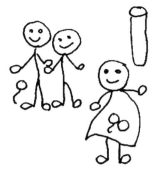

Gay male couple, traditional surrogate assisted pregnancy

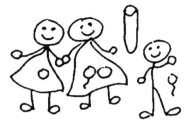

Lesbian couple, donor sperm assisted pregnancy

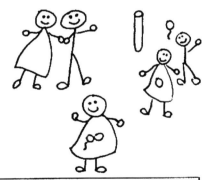

Donor embryo gestational carrier assisted pregnancy

participants in the fertilization and gestation process, yes. But they're neither the visionaries nor the creators of a new life and, to my mind, they should never be accorded the status of parents.

My Story: A Rocky Start

Unlike many of my fellow parents-through-technology, I've had a fairly easy time of it. I didn't have to endure the trauma of long-standing infertility. I didn't have to feel my marriage strain to the breaking point from years of sex on demand for the purpose of procreation. For me, the issue was age. Could I achieve a successful pregnancy again at 49? I didn't know, but I was excited by the challenge of trying.

My journey into ART actually began when I was nearly 48, with an unanticipated, spontaneous pregnancy. At the time, I had been experiencing approaching menopause, with hot flashes and all. So you can imagine my surprise when I learned, after I had missed a period, that I was pregnant. I was thrilled to discover my body could still give me such a gift. On the other hand, I knew from my medical training it was likely that I would miscarry because of chromosomal problems at my age. My fears were confirmed three weeks later when I saw by pelvic ultrasound that my embryo had, indeed, stopped growing.

In retrospect, I believe the loss of this pregnancy acted as my wake up call. I couldn't stop thinking about how wonderful it would have been to have had another child. A month later, while discussing my experience with an old friend (who happened to be an REI specialist), I began thinking seriously about how this dream might become a reality. My friend suggested that perhaps all my eggs were not too old and that I could try a cycle of in vitro fertilization with him to see if there were any viable eggs left. My hopes soared, in spite of myself.

After much discussion and consideration, David and I went to my friend's office in Chicago, to undergo an IVF cycle. Amazingly, in spite of my age, after a course of hormone shots to stimulate ovulation, 25 follicles arose within me. I felt like a mother hen, all bloated with my eggs. The retrieval went well. Eight eggs were successfully withdrawn. Then they were exposed to David's sperm—and we hit a snag. Through the embryologist's microscope, I could see that the eggs were trying to fertilize, but they were sluggish, doing their best to assert life, but to no avail. They were never going to make it. So with sadness and resignation, I let go of my hopes. I had felt so sure that there was a little egg just waiting inside me to be called out, to receive life. But now I knew there would be no pregnancy. So David and I returned to Hawaii, knowing we had tried our best.

On our way home, we stopped in Honolulu, where I had been invited to speak to a group of REI specialists and the embryologist at Honolulu's primary maternity hospital. Since they'd never met a 48-year-old woman who'd been stimulated for IVF, they were keen to hear what I had learned from my experience. The group listened, fascinated, as I explained what I'd seen under the microscope, the coarse, irregular chromatin of the nuclei and other details.

One REI specialist commented that clearly I was fit as a fiddle and that my uterus and hormonal system had behaved like a 25-year-old's, so certainly I could get pregnant if I went with a donor ovum.

David's reaction was typical of most men when the idea of using an ovum donor is first suggested. "Thanks, but no thanks. If it's not Lonny's egg, I'm not interested." I pretty much felt the same. We just weren't ready.

But the specialist didn't seem to be listening. She went on describing the many intelligent young women, including veterinary, medical, and engineering students, who were on her office's donor list, any of whom would be a great match for me. I laughed, thanked her, and then said with a smile, "Even if I were interested in ovum donation, I wouldn't care about having a 'brainy' egg. Good grief, I can educate any old egg on the brains from David's sperm alone. The qualities I'd look for would be those that would complement my husband's. Otherwise the poor kid would be a stick-in-the-mud."

I was hardly being serious. But I went on to say that I would want a woman who had had children already, so she would have an intrinsic understanding of the value of her gift to another woman, someone lively, with a great sense of humor, who loved animals, liked dining out and meeting others . . . someone like me. I also mentioned that I'd want someone with a healthy family medical history. I felt a high school education would be enough, if there were no learning disorders.

For me, the singularly most important factor would be my donor's willingness to be contacted in the future, if that were what I felt were in my child's best interests. I felt that any child of mine should have the option of knowing all about his or her roots, and it would be my responsibility as a parent to provide this opportunity at the right time.

Well, at this point, the discussion took an amazing turn. The REI specialist had been listening intently. Suddenly, she turned to a bookcase along the wall, pulled out an album, and held it out to me. "Someone like this?" she asked.

I leafed through the album. A woman who wanted to be a donor had compiled it. It began with a lovely handwritten note, in which she explained that she wanted to give another woman the happiness of creating a child, the gift of the miracle of life. She had a son; she included a picture of him as a toddler. She had been an A student in high school, but had chosen not to pursue college. She loved animals. She had several pets, adopted from an animal shelter. She loved to dance. Her parents were artistic. She enjoyed renovating old houses and doing stunt work for the movies. She would be happy to remain anonymous or to be contacted, but she would leave that decision up to the parents. She exhibited a clear sense of pride in her wish to be a donor. She mentioned that her sister had been a donor twice and had found the experience wonderful.

"Yup," I told the REI specialist. "If we were doing this, I'd pick her in a heartbeat."

But David and I still weren't interested. Instead, we were ready to accept my entry into menopause as the next natural step in our lives. After that meeting, we returned to the windward side of Oahu and I resumed my Ob/Gyn practice. We didn't talk about ovum donation again. Life went on.

Looking back now, I think I was somewhat in denial during this time about my desire to be a mother again. Logic told me I needed to give up this chapter of my life, but my heart said otherwise. Working underneath it all was a bit of depression from living in the empty nest. David and I both missed our older children, who were now grown and gone, and we realized it would probably be years before there would be grandchildren in our lives. It was far too quiet around the house, and although I tried, I just couldn't seem to accept the finality of menopause.

Then, eight months later, I received a message at my office to call back a woman whom I'll call "Kelly," who'd left a number. My staff and I looked for the patient's record, but we couldn't find it, and I didn't recognize the name. When I returned the call, Kelly introduced herself. "I am a donor candidate for a group of infertility doctors who work in Honolulu," she said. I felt a chill. I knew this was the woman who had created the album. And I knew what was coming next.

Kelly continued, "Last year before leaving to start a new practice, one of the infertility doctors told me about a female gynecologist in Oahu who would have been a perfect match for my egg, but wasn't interested in pursuing a donor. I've been thinking about that woman ever since. Are you the one? If you are, it would be an honor to give you my eggs."

I was in tears. "This is amazing," I managed to stammer. "Yes, I'm the one. How did you ever find me?" I went on to tell her how sweet and thoughtful I thought she was to have located me after all these months, but that I was content with the family I had. We talked some more, and I decided that despite my personal decision not to pursue a pregnancy, I'd still like to meet her. My patients with infertility often asked why I thought someone would want to be a donor, and I wanted to talk to her about that. "If I send you a plane ticket, will you come?" I asked. "Sure," she responded. She was on vacation on Kauai with her husband and son, and I sent her a ticket for a commuter flight to Oahu the following weekend right before Labor Day.

David and I went together to the airport to meet her. I recognized her right away—with a shock. We were dressed casually alike, in jeans, with our hair pulled up in scraggly topknots. She looked something like my daughter, too. We started laughing together at how similar our choices in style of clothing and hair-do were; it felt like a reunion.

The three of us spent the day at the small farm where David and I kept our horses. She'd never ridden before and wanted to try, so I put her on one of our horses and led her around the corral. We gabbed non-stop. Lunchtime came, and she pulled out of her handbag a family album she had brought with her. I couldn't believe it; I had brought ours too. Another coincidence. By the time we sat down to eat, poor David couldn't get in a word. He just watched and listened, often with a little half-smile on his face.

Kelly and I said good-bye at the airport with tears in our eyes. We talked about the paradox I was in. If I didn't follow through with Kelly's kind offer, then I would have met a lovely new friend whom I might see from time to time. But if I did go for it, and if I then developed misgivings about the wisdom of continuing a friendship after my child was born, I might never see her again. Revealing the truth about genetic roots to my child was one thing, but allowing my child to have a personal relationship with my donor was a much tougher decision. It was a decision that I knew should be based on what I believed would be best for my child, not on my own need to feel comfortable with my donor or my interest in having her as a friend. I thanked her for coming and said I hoped we would stay in touch, at least by letter.

When I returned to the car, I was in a state; it was all so overwhelming. "If I were to have a baby with a donor," I told David. "I'd want the donor to be Kelly and no one else."

"Before I saw the two of you together," he answered, "I couldn't imagine going for DE (donor egg). But you were like two sisters. If this is really what you want, I'd be willing to consider it."

I still wasn't ready, not without some more research. I began by looking for an infertility clinic that would match my needs. Since my uterus had previously grown two babies without complication, I didn't need a specialist in that area. But, obviously, I needed a clinic that was easy to get to from our home in Hawaii. More importantly, I wanted the facility's staff to include an experienced embryologist, someone with a good record growing embryos in vitro. I also wanted to be sure that the clinic I selected had a good track record with embryos surviving freezing and thawing, in case my first transfer weren't successful and I needed to try again.

I also needed my doctor—my REI specialist—to be easily accessible. I'd heard too many stories about couples who had spoken with their doctor at the initial interview and then never saw him or her again, except at the time of the actual transfer procedure. I wanted to know that my treatment would be handled directly by my doctor, and that he or she would be available to me when it was time to interpret lab results and make tough decisions.

My choice of a facility would also be influenced by the predominant policy during those years—this was in the early 1990's—regarding the anonymity of donors. Most clinics insisted on donor anonymity, but I felt, and I continue to feel, that the decision to know or not know a donor should be up to the prospective parents. If David and I decided on ovum donation, I wanted to know that the facility I selected shared my view about openness.

I approached several clinics, presenting myself as a woman in search of a donor. I was asked to fill out various questionnaires and was soon presented with a number of candidate profiles. None of them came anywhere near to feeling right for me. So, I called Kelly and asked whether she were still interested in donating her ova.

"Are you kidding?" she said. "Any egg of mine would be lucky to be given a chance for a life in a family like yours!"

The rest, as they say, is history. I finally found a clinic I liked. That was in the end of September. By Thanksgiving, my donor and I had synchronized our cycles, and we were ready to harvest her eggs, fertilize them with my husband's sperm and transfer them to me. By then, we all believed we'd be successful and that the new baby we were creating was simply meant to be.

The Secrecy Issue: Do You Want to Know your Donor?

Once the decision to move forward with Kelly's eggs was made, I began to think more about the whole subject of secrecy and communication between ovum donor and recipient. As the future mother of a baby created with donor ovum, I had more reason than ever to care about openness between donors and recipient families. Shortly after I selected the clinic that I would use for ART, I was interviewed by one of the clinic's social workers. She was emphatic that it would be better for everyone concerned if I used an anonymous donor, and she insisted that I was taking a considerable risk by selecting someone I had met recently who was neither a relative nor someone I knew well. She offered a few generalizations in support of her view, but she didn't seem interested in hearing why I wanted a donor who would be willing to meet my child should my husband and I decide that such a meeting would be appropriate. She didn't ask if Kelly and I had discussed how to handle any future disagreements that might arise over the kinds and frequency of contacts between the two of us, or between Kelly and my child, and she didn't suggest that we should consider having a written agreement to address such issues. She didn't suggest that my pre-ART views might change when I became pregnant or after delivery, nor did she remind me of the hormonally induced emotional swings that accompany pregnancy.

Looking back, it's hard to imagine how I went into such a significant life experience with so little professional guidance or support. I don't regret any of my choices, but I wish I'd known more, so that I'd have been better prepared emotionally. The one pre-retrieval psychological interview that I was given was hardly adequate and cannot have told the clinic much about me and my emotional needs.

Today there are a number of infertility books and web sites available to help families learn whether they might be good candidates for ART. But these resources still focus primarily on practical matters. Most fertility clinics still don't provide well-informed, ongoing emotional support as an integral part of their treatment programs. Instead, they refer patients to web site support groups or to outside counseling. I think this creates the impression that having worries and anxieties about ART is somehow abnormal. The ART system as a whole is still more geared to be reactive rather than pro-active; it doesn't really address common emotional needs. *Everyone* embarking on family building with technical assistance needs and deserves to have hand holding every step of the way.

Now I have to say one thing right here: The way I ended up with my donor was unique and still is. Kelly found me, not the other way around. It only happened as a result of an REI specialist making a mistake in breaking with complete confidentiality, accidentally revealing my profession, and a savvy potential donor who played detective and tracked me down. This unique circumstance meant that I began my ART experience with a known donor who was neither a relative nor a close friend nor even an acquaintance whom I had known for many years. But this sort of known donor is becoming more common. Except for the fact that our first contact was at Kelly's initiative, Kelly becoming a donor receptive to contact with a recipient family followed a familiar pattern. She knew someone who had been a donor (her sister) and had found the experience rewarding. Kelly had had a child of her own and felt empathy for those who were having trouble becoming mothers. She could envision her egg contributing to the making of a child that would be raised in a loving home by a loving couple, and she could envision having a healthy, non-threatening relationship with this child and couple as the child grew. Motivated to act by her empathy, and confident in what she imagined might result from her actions, she contacted a reproductive endocrinology and infertility (REI) clinic to offer herself as a donor and to express her willingness to have contact with the recipient family.

As I describe in Chapter 8, my experience with Kelly has been a wonderfully rewarding one. And Kelly has a warm friendship with my family. But during the early years, issues and questions arose along the way, particularly for me, and I had to work through those issues, and find answers to the questions, pretty much on my own. The REI clinic I selected was not prepared to help me anticipate the issues and questions that should be considered with third party assistance.

Even today, relatively few REI clinics are equipped to deal with special issues relating to the use of known donors. Some clinics that accept patients who express an interest in the use of a known donor make no efforts to screen for donor candidates willing to meet potential recipients in advance or willing to permit contact with a recipient family in the future. Even fewer clinics have counseling staff familiar with the emotional issues that can arise in connection with the use of a known donor with whom future contact is planned, let alone with the practical and legal issues.

One factor to consider in choosing a known vs. an anonymous donor is the accessibility of new medical information about the donor and his or her family years after an ART procedure. Such information may be needed to determine if a disease or condition developed by a DE, DI (donor insemination), or donor embryo child is hereditary and therefore likely to be passed on to the child's offspring. Most REI clinics consider donors to be clinic "patients" whose records must be retained for a legally mandated period of time. But if the clinic should close, or if the records should be lost due to fire or negligence, the required information may be lost or forever inaccessible. The Ethics Committee of the American Society of Reproductive Medicine (ASRM) urges REI clinics and sperm banks to consider how to preserve all records, including those of donors, if the clinic's REI specialist retires, or if the clinic or sperm bank closes.[14]

State laws differ on issues related to retention of medical records. Hawaii law, for example, allows medical records to be destroyed after seven years, although basic patient identifying information must be retained for 25 years.[15] Hawaii law also requires that agencies that place children for adoption "make reasonable efforts [to collect]

---

[14] Ethics Committee of the American Society for Reproductive Medicine, "Informing Offspring of their Conception by Gamete Donation," *Fertility and Sterility*, Vol. 81, No. 3, March 2004.

[15] Chapter 622, Section 622-58, Hawaii Revised Statutes.

information relating to the adopted child's potential genetic or other inheritable diseases or afflictions, including . . . known genetic disorders, inheritable diseases, and similar medical histories . . . ."[16] This law requires child placing agencies to "make reasonable efforts" to obtain written consent from the child's natural parents "to release this information to or for the benefit of the adopted child" and to obtain copies of the natural mother's medical records relating to the birth of the child.[17] However, there are no corresponding legal requirements imposed on REI clinics relating to children born through donor ovum or donor sperm ART.

Use of a known donor means that the recipient family will always be able to contact the donor to share new medical information and will not have to rely on the record keeping of a clinic. An ongoing relationship with a known donor also means that if a recipient family needs help from the donor that goes beyond the providing of medical information, that help may well be forthcoming. If, for example, a DE, DI, or donor embryo child were to develop leukemia and need a bone marrow transplant, the chances of finding a marrow donor with tissue compatibility would be enhanced if the potential marrow donors include the child's mother's ovum, sperm, or embryo donor or even a genetic full or half sibling (i.e., the child of the donor). And the donor might need this sort of help for his or her child sometime in the future; the request could come from either family. Such a request is far more likely to elicit a favorable response if the two families have stayed in contact and have a good relationship.

When One Door Closes, Another Opens

Monica, an infertile single woman, had tried without success to become pregnant using donor ovum and donor sperm. She decided to try again using donor embryos, but she wanted to use embryos from a known donor couple so that her future children would not

---

[16] Chapter 578, Section 578-14.5, Hawaii Revised Statutes.
[17] Ibid.

be isolated in a single-parent family, but could know the others who had been a part of their coming to life. She writes:

"My clinic had a number of ART families who had completed their childbearing and were offering their remaining embryos to other infertile women, but the clinic also had an absolute anonymity policy, which totally flew in the face of my values and put me in a difficult paradox," she explains. "My future children were available to me, but only if I were willing to deprive them of all access to their genetic heritage. How unreasonable it seemed! How unfair that the clinic should dictate a decision about disclosure that I felt was mine and should be based on my children's need to know."

Monica took her dilemma online, to Mothers Via Egg Donation (MVED), and received an unexpected response.

"A couple read my posting and e-mailed me privately to tell me that they had already had a child by anonymous donor ovum, their family was complete, and now they were experiencing the same issue I was from the other side of the fence. They had a number of frozen embryos that they wanted to donate, but their clinic also required anonymity. They were hesitant to agree to such a restrictive policy. They felt that their child might one day want to know any siblings who would be born if those embryos were brought to life."

Monica and the donating couple decided to take a leap of faith together.

"We began an e-mail correspondence, sharing our beliefs about the importance of disclosure of birth origins to children. And then we agreed to move ahead privately. There were no costs involved besides shipping and attorney fees. I, of course, paid my clinic for the procedure. It worked well for all of us; we have a very open line of communication, with contracts providing the boundaries of rights and expectations. It does not feel like an adoption because I carried the embryos and gave my twins life. I am their birth mother, even though my DNA was not part of the equation. But the circumstances are unique; there is a very warm and special link to the donating couple and my children's sibling. Our families stay in touch through mail and photos, and some day, when my children are ready, they will meet their sibling and their sperm donor."

Monica's story is unusual. She was able to circumvent her REI clinic's policy of requiring anonymous embryo donation by finding an embryo donor family on her own and reaching an understanding with that family that would allow future contact. She saw the biological male donor as someone with whom her own children might one day have a warm relationship, and she saw value in insuring that her children would have an opportunity to meet their full genetic sibling. I have no doubt that the bonds between the children in both families will be strong and enduring, not only because of their common genetic heritage, but primarily because of the shared values of their respective parents.

Ideally, all clinics storing embryos for couples that have completed their families should offer the option of what is sometimes called "willing-to-be-known" embryo donation/adoption. Many are not set up to do this, and they should be.

My Story Continues: A Surprise and a Tough Choice

Once Kelly's and my cycles had been synchronized, my REI clinic harvested a number of healthy eggs from her, and David's and my hopes mounted. It was likely that we would be creating many embryos. But on the day of my transfer, I learned that only six of the initial 10 embryos were thriving, and none of them were "top grade." (With many women, it isn't unusual to harvest 20 eggs, from which there might be 14 or more viable embryos). Because the embryos in my instance showed bits of debris outside the cells, my REI doctor wanted to facilitate the implanting. He asked me if I would agree to have the embryologist cut a tiny opening in the shell surrounding each embryo to help the cells escape to implant in the uterine lining, a procedure known as "assisted hatching." Then he wanted to place all six of the treated embryos inside of me, in the hope that at least one of them would be strong enough to implant and survive.

Remarkably, all of this was presented to me only moments before my transfer, as I prepared to lie on the table waiting for the procedure. I felt panicky. What if all six survived? How would I manage to raise that number of children? Then it hit me that I might not even survive such an unwieldy, multiple pregnancy, and I was really scared.

What if I delivered six babies? In spite of all the charming media stories about the arrival of quadruplets, quintuplets, sextuplets, and even septuplets, the reality is far more complicated; what you don't hear so much about are the challenges these parents confront. Babies from such higher order pregnancies are likely to deliver at 28 weeks or earlier and often have serious continuing health difficulties associated with premature births, including problems with breathing, cerebral hemorrhaging, and various neurological problems, as well as significant ongoing developmental delay.

Despite my last minute concerns, I followed my doctor's advice and had all six embryos transferred. Not everyone would agree with my doctor's advice, but in the end, he turned out to be right. Only one of the six embryos implanted, and this embryo resulted in a healthy, full-term birth, my son Tucker. The entire process, as well as the decision-making, would have been so much simpler and easier if just one or two embryos could have been transferred and had been able to survive. But science is not reliably there yet, so prospective parents may have to wrestle with the same issue I did. Specifically, you must decide, before you undergo embryo transfer, how many children you are willing to carry.

This is not an easy decision. Ideally you'll have some time before the transfer procedure to decide whether you're prepared to have a multiple pregnancy reduced through selective reduction if too many embryos "take." If you are not prepared to undergo selective reduction, then you must tell this to your doctor beforehand. If you do not want selective reduction and you are not prepared to risk carrying and delivering twins, triplets, quadruplets, etc., then you may want to ask your doctor to limit the number of embryos transferred. If this is what you decide, you must also be ready to accept that your chances for achieving pregnancy will likely decrease if fewer embryos are placed and/or their quality is less than ideal. And you may have to undergo multiple transfer attempts.

Your decision about how many embryos to transfer may also be affected by what stage the embryos have reached. For example, today, some clinic laboratories are able to nurture your embryos to the blastocyst stage (embryos that have thrived in the laboratory through five days post-retrieval). Back in 1995, we only had the option of transferring multiple three-day embryos since blastocyst cultures hadn't been reliably perfected. If your clinic has a greater than 50% success rate with fresh blastocyst transfers, it might be worth your transferring only one blastocyst at a time, since one of these sturdier, more advanced embryos would be more likely to implant. Even with blastocyst transfer, you need to be willing to undergo multiple attempts if you are clear about wanting only to carry a singleton pregnancy.

In addition to my concerns about carrying a higher order pregnancy and the increased risk to me or my unborn children, I also found myself thinking about what a multiple pregnancy would mean to our other children. By risking my health or life to carry more than one baby, I might also be depriving the children I had already been raising of the healthy mother they deserved.

With today's scientific sophistication, many people assume that operating rooms and intensive care units can handle any medical or surgical complication that arises for expectant mothers who are carrying more than one fetus. But this is not always the case. Hypertension, pre-eclampsia, coagulopathies (blood problems that place women at risk for hemorrhage), and diabetes, to mention some of the more common concerns, can still threaten the life of a woman carrying a higher order pregnancy. Even in singleton pregnancies, a modern tertiary care center provides no guarantees of a smooth ride.

Here's a sobering story posted to an on-line support group from a young mother following the delivery of her male twins at 28 and a half weeks:

Katie's Boys

The following is an e-mail I received from one of the women with whom I have corresponded about ART.

"I have read so many birth stories that have brought tears to my eyes and have always anticipated writing my own. I had no idea that it would not be the happy occasion I had envisioned—taking a few moments to write as my babies napped quietly by my side. Instead, as I write this, they are in the hospital intensive care unit, fighting for their lives."

The story . . .

"I am usually a good sleeper, but about three times a year I have insomnia. This night was one of them. At 12:30 AM, I felt a warm gush of fluid and thought I might have broken my waters or leaked some urine. I called the doctor, but I didn't hear anything back. Then I called my mom, who lives a half hour away, to come and watch our 3-year-old daughter. I really didn't think we'd have a birth that morning. Still, something made me feel the urgency of the situation, and my husband woke a neighbor to stand by until my mother arrived.

"The hospital was 30 minutes away. We sped off into the night and made the drive in 20 minutes. When we arrived, we learned that our doctor was just finishing a C-section. No wonder we hadn't heard from him. So the nurse checked me in, and I was immediately hooked up to a monitor and could see that the babies' heart rates were okay. Next, the resident doctor arrived and examined me. He said I was going to deliver soon. I asked about delaying the delivery and giving me steroids to help the babies' lungs develop, but was told that I had dilated too far to stop labor and there wouldn't be time for steroids to take effect.

"They wheeled me down to delivery, where our doctor was scrubbing up. Two teams of professionals were standing by to receive the babies. After a brief greeting, the doctor checked the fetal monitor, then got right to work, deciding to take the smaller, breech twin first. He was 2lbs 7 oz. I never heard him cry. They intubated him immediately to get his lungs working. Twin B came out a minute later. He was 3lbs 1oz. I watched as they intubated him and put in an umbilical line. The room was without a sound to be heard, just the bustle of professionals working quietly together. Before the babies were whisked to the neonatal intensive care unit, we had a chance to view them together in their mobile bassinet, among a tangle of IV lines.

"Later we were allowed into the NICU, after the babies were cleaned up and stabilized. They were larger than I'd anticipated. They were not fat and full like most newborns, but all their parts were there, even some hair. Baby A was having circulation problems; his feet were deep purple. Baby B was bigger, but his coloring was quite red. Whenever I put my finger into their small hands, they would grab at it. Pretty strong for such little guys. When I started to stroke and sing to each of them, the nurse told me kindly that this would over stimulate them. So I had to stop. We were allowed to cup head and feet together, containing each of them like they had been in the womb.

"These little boys were kicking and thrashing, which I thought was a good sign. But then I was informed that this was agitation, and they could pull out their respirator tubes and disrupt their lines, so their sedation was upped. They've been on heavy sedation ever since. For the first few days, they had lines running through their umbilical vessels that contained monitors and also gave them nutrients. These were removed a few days ago. Now they have lines in their arms.

"We've been told that they will probably remain in the NICU until their original due date. As for their condition, while it's not fatal, there have been many complications—lungs, heart, blood pressure, brain bleeds, temperature instability. There are many good stories about 28 weekers; I don't know if ours will be one of them."

Message to ART Professionals: What We Need to Do Differently

My experience with ART has made me acutely aware of all the shortcomings of the field. Changes are needed. Here's what I think should happen, and the sooner the better:

1) **REI clinics need to provide for better psychological support for their patients (including donors) and their partners.**

   Many clinics still do not have trained counselors on their staff and either gloss over the psychological and emotional issues raised by ART or send their patients to outside practitioners. Many clinics that offer counseling don't give it the emphasis it deserves or don't provide for continued support after a clinical pregnancy is achieved. Psychological support needs to be an integral part of the ART process at all REI clinics. A series of infertility management counseling sessions should be a mandatory part of the experience for any ART candidate and a recognized part of the clinic's treatment plan. Procedures must be carefully spelled out to patients, and the emotional consequences of upcoming choices fully examined by counselors trained in reproductive medicine. Patients need guidance in exploring what they believe about parenthood and how their beliefs might factor into the many decisions they will have to make. Couples need to talk about how authentic they'll feel as parents when genetic or gestational assistance has been necessary. They'll need to explore ways to cope with the esteem-crushing stresses that lie ahead. How are they going to deal with questions from family and friends? What will they tell their future children about ART? If there are siblings, what should they be told, and when? Patients should be provided a list of resources for pregnancy and post-partum support in their home area for when they return to their own doctor's care after ART.

2) **REI clinics need to do a better job of evaluating the efficacy of new procedures and tracking the long-term implications for the children of ART**

   I'm concerned that new procedures or variables in the evolving science of ART aren't being adequately studied and documented. For example, scientists should be studying and evaluating the effects of assisted hatching, ICSI, the changing of IVF growth media at various stages of embryo nurture, the use of intravenous gamma globulin to suppress embryo rejection, the administering of Viagra to women to enhance uterine lining, and a host of other facilitating procedures and treatments. These procedures and treatments should be evaluated not only with respect to their success rates in helping candidates achieve viable pregnancies, but also in terms of possible effects that may be passed on to offspring. We don't know what conditions might arise as these babies grow into adulthood and age. As yet, we have no systematized outcome surveillance in place for this first generation of ART children.

I think the REI specialist, obstetrician, and pediatrician should form a team to track long-term outcomes of every child so conceived or carried. The REI specialist should forward a summary of infertility treatments and manipulative procedures involving gametes and embryos to both the patient's obstetrician/gynecologist and the donor's gynecologist. The obstetrician should then be required to add comments pertaining to any complications during pregnancy and forward the records to the pediatrician, who would track the child to adulthood. Each physician involved in the ART family's ongoing health care would periodically enter health data into a national ART registry data base. In that way, we'd have the best chance of learning how our science is progressing.

A Tale of Two Consults

Here is another reminder of how important and meaningful the role of a counselor is for anyone undertaking the journey through the ART process.

In my friend Lucinda's own words:

"My experience with ART seems only to get more and more unpredictable as it goes along! Recently, I had two consultations, both with professionals and both with startlingly different and unpredictable outcomes.

"The first encounter was with a certified nurse midwife, supposedly one of the best in my large urban area, who works with the only hospital in the area to have an Alternative Birthing Center.

The Center is complete with water birthing suites, which makes my heart go pitter-pat in a big happy way. My husband and I had a consult with her a couple of years ago, when we were still optimistic about getting pregnant with my own eggs, and she was reassuring about my age (40ish) and my weight (200+ lbs) not being factors to label me 'high risk.' She said that as long as I could maintain a pregnancy until 38 weeks, I could have a low-tech, high-touch water birth in the Center. I've clung to that thought like an unclaimed winning lottery ticket ever since.

"But that initial consult with the midwife was before we met my immunologist and found out about all the little autoimmune gremlins hiding in my bloodstream. And it was before I knew I was carrying twins.

"My immune problems—and especially my long list of medications—totally freaked out the midwife. She asked what my doctor thought the effect of all of these medications would have on my pregnancy.

"Reading between the lines, I caught her real question: 'What doctor would be crazy enough to help you get pregnant with all these horrible problems?' I wonder what she would have said if I'd told her that my babies were created with donor ova and donor sperm to boot!

"She didn't seem to understand the difference between a reproductive endocrinology and infertility specialist (the IVF doc who created and transferred the embryos) and a reproductive immunologist (the specialist who treats my haywire immune system with blood tests and medications). She did say that, with twins, the Alternative Birthing Center was out of the question for me, and that she wanted me to see the Ob/Gyn in her practice. She said airily that if the OB doctor laughed her out of the room for bringing in such an impossible patient, she was sure he could refer me to a maternal-fetal medicine specialist who would be courageous enough to take my case.

"When I mentioned my concerns about my second twin measuring smaller and less proportionate than Baby A, she wrinkled her nose, shook her head, and said, 'Oh well, that second baby's not going to make it. Those measurements are just too screwy.' Then she brightened. 'Hey, but if you do wind up having a singleton, then you can go to the Alternative Birthing Center, after all. So everything might just work out for you and you'll have a singleton. Let's hope that's how it goes.' Is there a Hallmark card for this? 'Here's hoping your fetus dies so you won't be such a pain-in-the-butt of a patient?'

"By the time I left, I was good and truly frosted. My first cell phone call was to my husband, and he was so straightforward, seeing to the heart of the problem and offering the solution so plainly. He said simply, 'She's not the right one, then.' And he's right. No sense wasting energy getting all righteously indignant; just fire her and move on. I realize that I'll have to give up my dreams of a midwife-directed natural birth in a Jacuzzi. Even if I could find a midwife with a more appropriate bedside manner, I'd run too big a risk by not hiring some bigger guns to look after a twin pregnancy.

"I know that I'll probably face a much more regimented birth with an OB at the helm—possibly wielding a scalpel for a C-section—and definitely NOT an OB who has anything to do with that tactless midwife! Obstetric care brings another bevy of choices to make now that we know we have twins, but we've made it through our other choices so far. We can make it through this."

The second encounter is just as extraordinary in the opposite direction. Lucinda's story continues:

"After searching for years and enduring a series of temporary clergy, my small, liberal church has finally found a pastor who seems like a perfect fit. She's a white-haired dynamo with a grandmother's wisdom and a young woman's enthusiasm, a laser-keen sense of justice and a discerning wit. I had the feeling from the first time I met her that she could be both a safe haven and a challenging teacher in my life. It's not often that I run across that combination.

"For weeks I toyed with the idea of telling her our story—all of it. It was risky, but the more I thought of it, the more I realized that, if she were open to the positive side of our story, she could offer us a kind of support that counselors and doctors and even support groups couldn't, which we could certainly use. And if my revelation appalled her, at least, by pastoral oath, she couldn't go blabbing it all over the church. So I made the appointment.

"We talked for two hours. I told her the entire story of our marriage; my first pregnancy and miscarriage at 18 weeks; the long years of ART failure; and the eventual decision to use both egg and sperm donors to spare our children our genetic legacies, which include my autoimmune issues, my husband's progressive neurological disease, plus diabetes and obesity that run in both lines.

"The pastor was pensive at first. She said, 'Let me get this straight. Your doctor took an egg from another woman, fertilized it in a Petri dish with sperm from a donor, and transferred the resulting embryo to your womb.' I said that was right. 'So I am not genetically related to this child I'm carrying,' I explained. (I talked with her before we knew I was carrying twins.)

"'And neither is your husband,' she said.

"No, neither is he.

"She laid a hand to her collarbone and said, 'As curious as I am to get off into all the technical details of how this works, I have to take a moment to really take this in. My heart is just so full.' Then she took both my hands in hers, looked into my eyes, and said, 'I am just so blown away by the level of selflessness both you and your husband have exhibited to get here. You have created this child out of pure love. Your love for each other has made this child, beyond the bonds of genetics.'

"BINGO!

"She said that stories as extraordinary as this one were rare and precious and that she'd never heard a story exactly like ours. I was astonished that she 'got it,' so completely and so quickly, and to a much greater depth than any doctor or counselor I'd ever met, even the ones who specialized in ART!

"She told me about a service she'd done called 'The Wholly Family,' in which she invited several different kinds of families to share their stories with the congregation. The point was to illustrate that there is no such thing as an 'average family,' but that, instead, family is how we define it for ourselves. Yet she said that even she didn't have a category for us. 'You're not this child's genetic parents, you're not its adoptive parents, you're not its foster parents,' she said. 'You're just its parents. That's it. You can't apply any label to what kind of parents you are, because your bond is pure love. How extraordinary.'

"She said that she would stand behind us 100% on whatever and whenever we decided to tell the church community, but she did encourage me strongly to tell them at some point. She said that the chance of ostracism would be dramatically reduced if we told more of the back story, as I had told her, instead of just point-blank stating that our child came from donor gametes. She also said that there's always going to be someone who disagrees with and disapproves of us, while there will also be someone who suffers in silence who will be touched by our story and helped by it, though we may never know it. It is to that person, she suggested, that we owed the telling of our story.

"Food for thought: We're certainly not going to go storming the pulpit for a public revelation this Sunday, but with pastoral support that strong, the possibility of sharing our unique brand of joy with the rest of the church and having a positive outcome seems more attainable than I'd dreamed.

"I can't explain the feeling of relief I felt after I talked with her. I could not have imagined a better outcome to my revelation. In fact, before I talked with her, I couldn't imagine an outcome as good as what actually happened! After years of enduring well meaning but thoughtless remarks from clueless acquaintances, abrupt encounters with unfeeling medical personnel, and insults by that foot-in-mouth midwife among others, my faith in humankind begins to rekindle.

"One of the things I like about this pastor is that she closes every meeting, even with just two people, with a sacred poem or reading. Here is the poem she read to close our amazing conversation:"

Out of the Stars

Out of the stars in their flight, out of the dust of eternity, here have we come,
Stardust and sunlight, mingling through time and through space.
Out of the stars have we come, up from time;
Out of the stars have we come.
Time out of time before time in the vastness of space, earth spun to orbit the sun,
Earth with the thunder of mountains newborn, the boiling of seas.
Earth warmed by sun, lit by sunlight:
This is our home;
Out of the stars have we come.
Mystery hidden in mystery, back through all time;
Mystery rising from rocks in the storm and the sea.
Out of the stars, rising from rocks and the sea,
kindled by sunlight on earth, arose life.
Ponder this thing in your heart; ponder with awe:
Out of the sea to the land, out of the shallows came ferns.
Out of the sea to the land, up from darkness to light,
Rising to walk and to fly, out of the sea trembled life.
Ponder this thing in your heart, life up from sea;
Eyes to behold, throats to sing, mates to love.[18]

---

[18] Responsive Reading #530 from the Unitarian hymnal "Singing the Living Tradition," published by Beacon Press, Boston, for the Unitarian Universalist Association, copyright 1993.

Chapter 4

Gifts From the Heart: The Other Partners in Your ART Experience

The science of ART is amazing, marvelous, miraculous. But so, too, are the people who agree to give of themselves, deeply and profoundly, to help an infertile couple create the family their hearts' desire.

Often, a third and even fourth person will be intimately, if not directly, involved in helping a couple become parents. Who are these wonderful, necessary, and compassionate people who donate sperm or eggs? Why do they give as they do? And, for the infertile couple, what does it feel like to have such close partners in a process that until recently involved only a man and a woman and a very private act? Let's take a look at the personal side of what is called third party assisted reproduction.

Sperm and Egg Donation

There's a lot to think about when receiving donor sperm and/or ova. When you go this route, you can have a gestational connection to your children without having made a genetic contribution. Under such circumstances, prospective parents may face unique emotional issues, as well as powerful cultural biases.

Sperm donation has been around for years and is generally accepted by our culture. Ovum donation, on the other hand, is newer and more controversial. Why is that? Perhaps it's just the newness. Or perhaps society attributes more importance to eggs because they are less plentiful and less accessible than sperm. The procedure for harvesting ova is quite invasive, too. Sperm are merely collected from ejaculate, while eggs are retrieved by inserting an ultrasound probe, which includes a hollow needle, into the vagina. Guided by the probe, the needle is inserted through the back wall of the vagina to reach the ovaries where eggs are extracted via aspiration. Perhaps if millions of eggs were passed out of the woman's body at each monthly period, as sperm are in an ejaculate, or perhaps if new eggs were continually made throughout the reproductive years as sperm are, the ovum would also come to be viewed as a more commonplace body product.

The reasons for the unequal attitudes about sperm versus ovum donation may also go deeper. I suspect some people find it easier to accept the notion of sperm donation because sperm can be cryopreserved intact without the need to be fertilized first. Until recently, the only way to preserve an ovum was for it to be fertilized. For those who believe that life begins at conception, this introduces the uncomfortable idea of holding human life in limbo. In the future, if more reliable results from cryopreserved ova and/or ovarian tissue are achieved, the concept of life in limbo won't be an issue. But until cryopreservation techniques are further refined and more consistent results achieved, I would not advise a patient to rely on cryopreservation of unfertilized ova if she is intending to delay childbearing.

Although society as a whole appears to be more comfortable with the idea of sperm donation than ovum donation, I have found that attitudes of couples and individuals struggling with infertility vary widely on this subject. Some partners are quite comfortable with the idea of ovum donation but are troubled by the idea of sperm donation. Sometimes a husband whose wife is infertile will confide that he would have preferred to have a child via sperm donation rather than use donated ova, while his wife expresses the opposite bias.

When I counsel patients on this subject, I offer three thoughts. First, I suggest that they take with a large grain of salt any comments made about either sperm or ovum donation from individuals, especially relatives and close friends, who have not had to confront infertility and make decisions about donor assistance for themselves. No one who looks at this subject in the abstract can predict how he or she would feel if faced with a real decision about his or her own children. Second, I point out the simple reality that egg and sperm make equal genetic contributions. After all, neither is going to get far without the other! Finally, I suggest that we all come with biases. It is not wrong to have a bias. But it *is* wrong to lose sight of the fact that every couple seeking to become parents through donor assistance is providing, entirely on its own, the most critical ingredients needed to create a child: love and commitment.

Who is the Parent? Psychological and Legal Issues

When a third or fourth person enters the picture and participates in helping an infertile couple bear a child, a host of questions arise regarding parentage. Our society is just beginning to address those questions. My own personal experience with ART has given me the opportunity to study and reflect at length on what exactly a parent is. The way I see it, there are four key elements involved in parenting:

1. Pre-conception psychological orientation and commitment;
2. Genetic contribution at conception;
3. Pre-delivery nurturing during gestation, both direct and indirect; and
4. Post-delivery nurturing.

I have listed these in chronological order (i.e., the order in which they either first arise in a prospective parent or first impact a child), not in order of importance. I have an opinion about their relative importance, but before I offer it, I want to describe each element in some detail.

By "pre-conception psychological orientation and commitment," I mean the mental and emotional preparation for parenthood that starts for all of us when we are infants—when we have parenting behavior first modeled for us by our own parents—and that continues through adolescence and on into our adult years, right up until the moment that our own children are conceived. I also mean the desire to have children and the willingness to make sacrifices in order to become a parent.

Our psychological and emotional readiness to be a parent, and our enthusiasm for this most important of all human endeavors, are determined to some degree by the way we ourselves were parented. If we were loved and nurtured and thoughtfully taught by our parents, we will be better prepared to be good parents ourselves, and we are more likely to want to be parents. Of course, growing up in a happy family with loving parents is by no means a guarantee that one will make a good parent. Nor is it a necessity; there are many wonderful parents whose own childhoods were very difficult. But few would dispute that exposure to good parenting in one's own family is highly desirable preparation for raising a family.

The meaning of "genetic contribution at conception" should be obvious. There are two genetic contributors to every child, the male contributor whose sperm fertilizes the ovum, and the female contributor whose ovum is fertilized. Note that I do not refer to these contributors as "genetic parents" or as the "genetic father" and "genetic mother." I prefer the terms "genetic contributor" or "genetic donor" because I believe the concept of parenthood involves so much more than the passing on of genes.

Pre-delivery nurturing during gestation includes both physiological and emotional nurturing, although the line between the two is somewhat blurred, in my view. It can also be either direct or indirect nurturing. I refer to the physiological and emotional nurturing of a fetus during gestation as "direct" nurturing when it is provided by the woman carrying the fetus, and I refer to it as "indirect" when it is provided by someone else.

A woman who undergoes IVF using a donor ovum and who carries and delivers her child provides direct pre-delivery nurturing during gestation. She nurtures her child in utero physiologically both by what she does (e.g., eating healthy foods, exercising sensibly, and getting plenty of rest) and what she avoids doing (e.g., smoking, drinking alcohol). And she nurtures her child emotionally by avoiding stress inducing activities or situations and by taking care of her own emotional needs. The environment she provides for the life growing within her will influence her child in a multitude of ways that science is only just beginning to understand. The influences on this environment—nutritional, chemical, auditory, kinesthetic, emotional—can range from the possibly trivial (e.g., attending loud rock concerts; listening to Mozart on the stereo; riding on a roller coaster; going sailing) to the potentially catastrophic (e.g., drinking heavily during the first trimester.)

This woman's partner can also have an important influence on his child's gestational environment. If he is attentive and supportive and understanding during the pregnancy, helping his wife do the best job she can nurturing their child during gestation, he will be a significant, albeit indirect, contributor to that nurturing.

In the case of a couple that uses a gestational carrier or traditional surrogate, the gestational carrier or traditional surrogate is the one providing the direct nurturing, but the parents who will raise the child can both have an important indirect influence on the child's prenatal environment. In addition to the financial support that ensures that the carrier or surrogate will receive good pre-natal care, eat well, and get adequate rest, they can provide critical emotional support. Most women who volunteer to become gestational carriers or surrogates are motivated not by the prospect of financial compensation, but by the idea that they will be helping an infertile couple become loving parents. They find the experience to be joyful and emotionally rewarding, and I have no doubt that this fact has important beneficial consequences for the child. Accordingly, all prenatal contacts that the future parents have with the carrier or surrogate that reassure her that she is helping a responsible, loving couple are contacts that directly support the carrier or surrogate and indirectly nurture the child in utero.

Of course, this same concept of indirect gestational nurturing applies in cases of adoption when a pregnant woman who intends to give up her child to adoption meets the adopting couple early in the pregnancy. Although I cannot cite any studies to support the idea, I believe that a woman carrying a child that she intends to give up for adoption will have a less stressful pregnancy, and will therefore provide her child with a more nurturing in utero environment, if she knows that her child will be raised by a responsible, loving couple. And this couple provides direct support to the birth mother, and therefore indirect support or nurturing to the unborn child, by reassuring the birth mother that the child she conceived and will deliver will have the advantages that come with being raised by loving parents.

Post-delivery nurturing, needless to say, includes all the love, support, and guidance that parents provide from the moment of birth through childhood, adolescence, and on into adulthood. It encompasses all of the words and the deeds and the sacrifices that parents make during a lifetime of interaction with their children.

How do I see the relative importance of these four elements involved in parenting? The last of the four, post-delivery nurturing, is in my opinion clearly the most important and the only one of the four that is absolutely necessary for one to deserve to be called a "parent." It is also the only one of the four that is sufficient, standing alone, to convey "parenthood" on an individual. Pre-conception psychological orientation and commitment alone is not enough. (An infertile woman that yearns for a child but that never conceives, adopts, or successfully undergoes some form or ART will, sadly, never be a parent.) Nor is direct pre-delivery nurturing during gestation enough. (A woman who delivers a baby that is adopted anonymously at birth is usually referred to as the child's "birth mother," but she will have no parental rights, parental responsibilities, or parental role in relation to that child after the adoption.) What about genetic contribution? Again, I do not think it can ever be enough, standing alone, to confer the status of "parenthood." An anonymous sperm donor is an important participant in the creation of a child, but what has that participation to do with the concept of "parenting" or of being a "father" to that child?

What about the relative importance of the first three elements of parenthood: pre-conception psychological orientation and commitment; genetic contribution at conception; and pre-delivery nurturing during gestation, both direct and indirect? Ranking these elements is a matter of personal opinion. I am unaware of any scientific research that would support one ranking over another. But I do believe, based on my understanding of genetics, which I summarize below, that genetics tends to be overemphasized, and both pre-conception psychological orientation/commitment and pre-delivery nurturing during gestation are often underrated or even overlooked.

Why do I bother to analyze parenthood in this way, breaking it down into four elements? I do it to explain how exceptional ART parents are as a group and why, as a general rule, they make wonderful parents.

If all parents were divided into three groups: ART parents, adoptive parents, and all other parents, one could make some useful, comparative generalizations about these three groups through reference to the four elements of parenting. With respect to the first element, pre-conception psychological orientation/commitment, it is clear that *all* ART parents and *all* adoptive parents become parents only as a result of a strong, thoughtful, and prolonged commitment to parenthood. Both the ART procedures and the legal requirements for adoption entail a substantial expenditure of time, effort, and money before dreams of parenthood can be realized. This expenditure is clear evidence of both a psychological orientation, as well as a commitment, to parenthood. Of course, most parents who become parents through intercourse, rather than via adoption or ART, also come to parenthood with a "pro-child" pre-conception orientation and commitment, but there are also many in this group who become parents via an unplanned pregnancy, as a result of failed birth control or unprotected sex. (I am not suggesting that such parents will not be good parents, merely that they cannot claim membership in an exclusive group *all* of whose members can point with pride to the sacrifices they have made to become parents.)

One can also make a valid, and I believe useful, generalization about ART parents with respect to the third element of parenting, pre-delivery nurturing during gestation. *All* ART parents contribute, either directly or indirectly, to the nurturing of their children during gestation. ART mothers via ovum donation, sperm donor insemination (DI), intracytoplasmic sperm injection (ICSI), gamete intrafallopian transfer (GIFT), and zygote intrafallopian transfer (ZIFT), all provide direct nurturing of their children during gestation, and their husbands or partners provide indirect nurturing. The ART parents of children born via traditional surrogate or gestational carrier all provide indirect nurturing of their children during gestation. This is because the process of arranging for a surrogate or gestational carrier invariably involves personal contact between parents and surrogate or carrier and ideally leads to the developing of close personal relationships among all parties.

By contrast, parents via anonymous adoption do not have the opportunity for indirect nurturing during gestation, and many parents via open adoption also lack this opportunity.[19] Nor can a generalization be made about the indirect nurturing available from fathers of children conceived via intercourse. A significant number of women who conceive, bear, and deliver their children will have no contact whatsoever with the men who fathered their children.

Why do I make these comparisons and regard them as "useful?" I make them because I think that many ART parents have bought into widespread, pre-ART views of parenthood as a status that is based primarily on one's genetic link to a child, but that is susceptible to redefinition by the courts on the basis of a commitment to nurture,

---

[19] Open adoption is a term that covers a wide range of options. Some open adoptions involve extensive contact between the birth mother and the adoptive parents. Others involve only an exchange of letters or personal information that is monitored and managed by the adoption agency.

historically through an adoption proceeding. This simplistic view places too much emphasis on genetics, in my opinion, and it fails to recognize and honor what is truly unique and wonderful about ART parents: the commitment, love, and sacrifice that they all invest in making the journey to parenthood, starting long before their child is conceived.

Keeping the foregoing discussion of parenthood in mind, let's look at some examples of contradictory, paradoxical, or just plain muddy thinking about parenthood reflected in our social institutions, particularly the courts.

Justina and Mark: Using a Gestational Carrier

Justina had a hysterectomy due to cervical cancer, but her ovaries still carried viable eggs. Once she passed the five-year mark without recurrence of her cancer, she and her husband, Mark, decided they were ready to start a family. Their close friend, Emily, whose family building was complete and whose fallopian tubes had been tied, offered to carry their child for them. She would be a gestational carrier for Justina and Mark. Justina's egg and Mark's sperm were joined in the laboratory through IVF, and the resulting embryo was transferred to Emily's womb. The embryo transferred to Emily was genetically Justina's and Mark's. It grew into a fetus and, after nine months, was delivered into the world by Emily as a beautiful, healthy baby girl.

Isn't it obvious that Justina and Mark are this baby's parents? They had the intent to create their child, and they had the intent and commitment to nurture it to adulthood. Yet, legally, in most states, Emily—the gestational carrier—would be automatically listed on the birth certificate as the baby's mother. And Justina would need to arrange *to adopt her own genetic baby*, or obtain a court order before the birth to be listed on the baby's birth certificate as the baby's mother. Ironically, Mark wouldn't need to go through those gyrations. According to the courts, his genetic contribution is enough to make him the baby's father. Not so for Justina when there is a gestational carrier involved.

Elaine and Arthur: Using an Ovum Donor

When Elaine and Arthur decided to have a baby together, they discovered that Elaine had no viable eggs. So Elaine selected a donor who was happy to provide some. The contract between the donor and Elaine and Arthur stated that the donor would give up all rights to the eggs that were retrieved and that the recipients would assume full responsibility for those eggs and any viable embryos that resulted. Following in vitro fertilization of the eggs with Arthur's sperm, two embryos were placed in Elaine, one of which survived, and nine months later Elaine gave birth to a healthy baby. Elaine and Arthur are listed on the birth certificate as the baby's parents. Would anyone doubt that they actually are this baby's parents, despite the lack of a genetic contribution from Elaine? Elaine and Arthur had the intent to create, bear and rear a child, not the donor. Yet some counselors and other so-called experts might say, in this instance, that the donor should be considered the child's genetic mother because she provided some of the genes to the process. Recall, however, that in the legal arena, genetics as a basis for parenthood is ignored in favor of gestation. Unless Justina, from the first example, adopted her own daughter, she would have no legally recognized relationship with her daughter. Paradoxically, in Justina's case the law says gestation rules, while in Elaine's case other professionals would say that genes rule. Ridiculous!

To further add to the confusion, not only may a psychologist's point of view be very different from a lawyer's or a judge's, but the definition of parent varies widely among families of different ethnicities and cultures.

Arlene and Faith: Using Both Ovum and Sperm Donors

Arlene and Faith, a lesbian couple, had been together for eighteen years. They had an eight-year-old adopted daughter, Katie, and decided they wanted to try for a sibling for their daughter using ART so their family could experience childbirth. Because both women were in their mid-to-late forties, they needed an ovum donor and a sperm donor. Together, Arlene and Faith selected the donors and decided that Faith, the younger of the two, would carry the pregnancy. Does anyone doubt that Arlene and Faith will be this baby's parents? Although the individual germ cells were not created by the parents in this instance, the child was. Arlene and Faith are the only ones, in fact, who had the intent to create, gestate and raise the child. How could the donors be considered genetic "parents," when they had no intention to be a part of this child's life beyond independently contributing some genes?

Another possible scenario that is fraught with legal problems is when one partner in a lesbian couple wants to "donate" her eggs to the other partner who will then carry the child so they both may participate in the process. This brings up issues of co-parenting, adoption, etc. Anyone considering any of these options should consult with professionals in all areas that will effect decisions along the way.

The Hearts and Minds of the Donors

A donor may not be called a parent, but his or her contribution is unique and irreplaceable. It's natural to want to know what kind of man or woman offers such a gift—and why. Here are some personal accounts from sperm and ovum donors.

Mariah, Ovum Donor: A Big Honor for a Small Role

"I appreciate your gratitude for the small contribution I made to your creating your twin daughters," Mariah writes in response to a thank you letter from her recipient family. "I am very honored that you chose me to serve as your donor. I do realize that my contribution was real, but I also know how minute my role was. I am myself the mother of two daughters and a son, and I know full well that it is taking care of them and loving them every day as they grow that makes them our children, not the genetics."

Jori, Ovum Donor: Passing on Special Qualities

"The reason I would like to do this," writes this 23-year-old graduate student, "is because I feel that I have a gift that some do not, of being able to have children. I want to help someone fulfill her dreams. I'm not in a serious relationship and I don't know whether I'll have children. In the meantime, by becoming a donor I can know that some of my special qualities will be passed on, enjoyed and appreciated."

Rose-Marie, Ovum Donor: Influenced by Adoption

"My parents adopted me because they couldn't have children any other way. My mom's and my relationship is what made me think about becoming a donor. I am so much a part of her life, and she is so much a part of mine. I'm married now with two wonderful children of my own. Whenever I watch them climb all over Gram's lap, clamoring for yet another story, I remember what it felt like to nestle in her arms when I was little, feeling so safe. By being a donor, I feel I'm giving out some of my mother's and my good fortune to others. Maybe my recipient will even be someone a little like my mom."

Melinda, Ovum Donor: Inspired by Nature

"I'm a marine biologist, and I've always been fascinated by the way nature seems to provide plenty of opportunity for survival of the young. I remember sitting on the beach, already a mother of four, and watching in fascinated silence as hundreds of tiny turtles emerged from their nests and then struggled across the sand to the safety of the sea. I thought about the abundance of life still within me, and that's when I first considered becoming a donor. My husband and I were very fortunate to have our children young; by the time we were 28, we had four kids. I had to have my tubes tied or start my own soccer team! As a woman and mother myself, I know the preciousness of the abundance my husband and I received. My eggs are great. Why waste them?"

Peter, Sperm Donor: Touched by Tragedy

"I was a pediatric resident and was deeply affected by one of my admissions. Actually, it was a re-admission: a little girl returning with leukemia. She was unlikely to survive this hospitalization. Her parents were so exhausted, but they were holding up well considering what lay ahead. I thought about my family, a pretty healthy bunch. What a contrast. I knew from my patient's family history that the dad had recently undergone radiation treatments for prostate cancer, rendering him sterile. It was likely this daughter would remain their one and only child. Learning that, I thought: wouldn't it be nice to be a donor for him, or someone like him, one day, when all the pain and sorrow of his daughter's death might have lessened enough to let him think he could be a parent once again? Right then, helping them handle their latest crisis, was all I could focus on. But that was when the idea of becoming a donor became a part of me. I am married now, a father of three and, with my family's blessing, have donated twice for cancer survivors."

Kami and Sam, Embryo Donors: Sharing the Bounty

"Sam and I have been truly blessed," writes Kami. "I have a genetic problem that means my ovaries can't make eggs. We had made our peace with that. Then, imagine how stunned we were after twenty-five years of marriage when the 1980's brought news of donor eggs."

"Now, thanks to ovum donation, we have twin daughters, age seven, and a son, age two. After our last pregnancy, we still had eight frozen embryos left. Our family was complete—we really didn't feel we could handle eight more children! After thinking long and hard, we decided to give the embryos a chance at life by finding parents who would really appreciate the miracle of such a gift. We were so lucky—our agency found a great match in another couple who wanted to adopt our embryos."

Receiving Donor Genes and Mourning the Lost Genetic Link

For most parents, using donated ova, sperm, or both, raises a host of feelings. It's natural to need to grieve the loss of a genetic link.

"Dealing with the genetic piece of the puzzle has unique meaning for every couple," says Judith Kottick, an experienced infertility counselor who has helped many women and men as they struggle with the decision to accept third party assistance in becoming parents. "For some recipients, family lineage is a larger part of their identity than they ever appreciated, until they were faced with it being taken away. In some families, there are certain traits, whether physical, temperamental, intellectual, or something else, that bonds the family in some profoundly meaningful way. I have heard such moving stories from people who express a profound sadness at the idea of being unable to pass down the potential for one trait or another . . . and sometimes it's something that to me might seem small and insignificant, but to them is enormous. Even if their child didn't end up having this trait, at least the potential exists. In other families, this is not the case—and these recipients are often less moved by the genetic piece, feeling more connected to the environment in which they grew up."

Kottick sees her task as helping couples come to terms with what genetics means to them and honoring their beliefs. "I don't try to talk them out of feeling, for instance, that genes are significant, but help them mourn what they have lost," she says. "I try to help all couples think about nature and nurture as a partnership, encouraging those who are most concerned with genes to remember the importance of nurture . . . and reminding those who are casual about genes not to dismiss the importance of the genetic contribution. I often ask couples to tell me about any siblings they may have—how are they alike and different. This is a great way to help them recognize the constant interplay of genetics and environment. I also think it's very hard for the yet-to-be parent to fully comprehend the profound impact of the parent-child bond. Without understanding that experience, recipients have no choice but to focus on the information they *do* have. So many times, what I hear from recipients once they have children is that the things they were so worried about seem so unimportant later. But there's no way to know that until you find out in real time!"[20]

In my own experience of accepting donor eggs, I found comfort and reassurance in learning more about the relevant science—what genes are and what they do and don't do. Most people assume that making a genetic contribution to a child is the same as carrying on their unique family tree of traits and talents. But is the genetic tapestry of their family so unique? It may not be as clear-cut as we suppose. In spite of what many believe, genes are not owned by individuals as if they were items of unique family furniture. In fact, scientists will tell you that all of mankind's DNA varies less than 1% from person to person. In other words, we all contain mostly identical family furniture. The genetic tapestry of a family is dramatically altered when genes (DNA) from two individuals are brought together in offspring. The relatively small number of differences among our tens of thousands of genes can combine in a mind bogglingly large number of ways.

In addition to this well-spring of diversity residing in the substance of our genes, the environments in which union of egg and sperm happen, and in which the embryo subsequently develops, influence the turning on or off processes that control the *expression* of genes.

It is amazing to think that from such a unity of nearly identical genetic building blocks we are able to have such immense diversity of expression. But that is where the environment combined with the random mixing of genetic information from different germ cells comes into the picture, turning off the making of messages in some instances, and in other instances modulating them to ignore one set of instructions for another, and so forth and so on from the moment an

---

[20] Author's personal correspondence with Judith Kottick, LCSW, a consultant to reproductive endocrinologists and attorneys in the Northeast, specializing in gestational surrogacy and egg donation. She also maintains a private counseling practice in Montclair, New Jersey.

embryo starts to form. This process of adaptation and specialization continues throughout the life of the organism.

New York Times Science writer and Pulitzer prize winner, Natalie Angier, writes eloquently about the subjugation of DNA to control by environmental forces in a 2003 New York Times article, *Not Just Genes: Moving Beyond Nature vs. Nurture*. "DNA on its own, does nothing. It can't make eyes blue, livers bilious or brains bulging. It holds bare bones information—suggestions, really—for the construction of the proteins of which *all* [my emphasis] life forms are built, but that's it. DNA can't read those instructions, it can't divide, it can't keep itself clean or sit up properly—proteins that surround it do all those tasks . . . ." Angier continues, "Nowhere is an appreciation for the perpetual crosstalk between gene and scene more important, these scientists say, than in understanding human nature. Loose talk about genes 'for' neurotic or novelty seeking behavior, sexual orientation or schizophrenia is misguided, not only because such language neglects the surely multigenic nature of nearly all characteristics worth studying, but because the phrase that puts genes at the command post ignores the ineluctably packaged, interactive deal that is DNA and its setting at every stage of life."[21]

As Dr. Martha McClintolk, professor of biopsychology at the University of Chicago, also comments, quoted in the same article: "There's a constant back and forth between genes and the environment. It's important to remember that genes came to be what they are solely because of their capacity to interact with the environment, and make the right products in response to the environment."[22]

I come away from this kind of examination realizing why it doesn't pay for me to get too carried away on the genetic issue. The genes that exert their effect in any given family are the same genes we find exerting their effects in all the family of man. This may be

---

[21] Natalie Angier, "Not Just Genes: Moving Beyond Nature vs. Nurture," *New York Times*, 25 Feb. 2003. Copyright © 2003 by the New York Times Co. Reprinted with permission.

[22] Ibid.

small comfort for the father who would like to create his child in his own image, but hoping to create a mini-version of himself through his children could actually be quite limiting for both parent and child, as every parent of a rebellious teenager knows! Children need to live out their own gifts and goals, not fulfill a parent's specific, tailor-made dream—one involving a preconceived idea of the role their genes should play.

There is another aspect of the scientific picture I also find illuminating. After the original egg-sperm union, it's the nutrients from the womb that increasingly supply all the components for making every new generation of cells. Those cells themselves, using building materials from the mother, create the substance of the growing baby's rapidly multiplying cells, including the genes. After the sperm penetrates the wall of the ovum, there is nothing left of the initial sperm's individuality as an independent cell. What once was two germ cells becomes an entirely new cell, containing enough genetic information to form a future embryo. In a Petri dish, this first cell, called a zygote, will undergo a single subdivision into two daughter cells. Then those two daughter cells will divide into four cells, then eight, and so forth and so on, until the cell bundle, a pre-embryo, is ready to be transferred into the womb.

The initial fertilized cell (zygote) that had undergone those first few cell divisions in the Petri dish before being placed in the womb has long since been replaced, after transfer, by generations of daughter cells, now entirely composed of nutrient materials from the mother. Only their pattern of instructions persists from the original merger of DNA. The resulting baby, including all the building blocks that make up its DNA, is more the mother's in substance than she realizes! Thus, it is clear that the contribution of a life-giving cell is not synonymous with the gift of a baby made up of someone else's cells. By the time a donor assisted ART baby is born, that first cell with its original foreign materials has long since ceased to exist.

Another way of making this same distinction is to think about baking a cake. If I were to receive a wonderful recipe from my sister for a cake that I wanted to make, first I would go out to the store and buy all the ingredients in the recipe. Then I would return home and put those ingredients together according to the instructions in the recipe. Having baked this cake in my oven, I might plan to serve it at a dinner party. People would marvel at my wonderful cake and perhaps comment on what a great recipe I had used, but in no one's mind would there be any question as to whose cake it was. In other words, a recipe cannot a cake make without the baker, her oven, her intent, and her ingredients.[23]

Still, there are difficulties to face when we can't follow the usual route to becoming a parent. And what happens when couples have to face an unequal genetic contribution? Let's take a look at ovum or sperm donation from the recipient's point of view.

Fathers and Donor Sperm

Fathers who need the help of a sperm donor face a system still shadowed by the legacy of sperm donation in the 1950's. At that time, there were some odd practices that seemed to imply there was something adulterous or shameful about receiving sperm donation. For example, semen from the husband was mixed with semen from the donor before the insemination, presumably to help maintain a fantasy that it was the husband's sperm that reached the egg, despite the fact that testing had indicated that the husband's sperm were not viable. Also, couples were encouraged to have intercourse after the insemination for the same reasons. It was as if doctors were trying to create a fictitious ambiguity in order to compensate fathers for their lost self-esteem and connection to fatherhood.

---

[23] For an excellent discussion of genetics, suitable for children as well as adults, see Mahlon Hoagland and Bert Dodson, *The Way Life Works: Everything You Need to Know About the Way Life Grows, Develops, Reproduces, and Gets Along*, (New York: Time Books, Random House, 1995). Dr. Hoagland is a noted molecular biologist best known as discoverer of amino acid activating enzymes and co-discoverer of transfer RNA, key elements in the translation of genetic information into living substance.

Thank goodness the medical community now has more sense. Yet the history of secrecy surrounding donor insemination (DI) has left a legacy. Only recently have some sperm banks begun to make information about the sperm donor available to prospective parents the way ovum donation resources have done.

Still, even today, with more information available in the selection of a sperm donor, a father may experience a kind of emotional disconnect, feeling his wife actually is carrying another man's baby. I suspect men in this situation may be subconsciously confusing the in vitro process with the act of lovemaking. But it must be remembered that the child his wife is carrying exists only because of his and his wife's shared desire to create new life and build a family together. It is wholly his and her baby—the sperm donor has played no role in the initiation and sharing of this vision.

Of course, a father who has not contributed his sperm to a successful pregnancy may still need to grieve the loss of his genetic contribution. As one father expressed to me, there is keen disappointment when the qualities in himself that he believed drew his wife to him in the first place might not be there for her to experience in their children.

Dr. Elizabeth Grill, an infertility counselor with the Center for Reproductive Medicine and Infertility at Weill Medical College of Cornell University, comments that "in addition to generalized anxiety in response to male factor infertility, men also struggle with the societal stigma of impotency, loss of genetic continuity for their family line, and poor self-esteem. Women may not understand the shame a man who associates potency with manliness may feel when he can't 'make' his wife pregnant."[24]

The coping mechanisms for a man may be different than for a woman. Even when there is male factor infertility, the woman may still have to go through numerous and often painful and invasive procedures to achieve a pregnancy. Dr. Grill goes on to say, "A failure of any kind has the potential to throw her into days of depression.

---

[24] Author's conversation with Dr. Elizabeth Grill

The husband, on the other hand, may feel overwhelmed by his wife's despair and her desire to talk about the infertility constantly. He may either respond with calm, reason, and optimism, in an effort to comfort his partner and be the strong one or he may feel like a failure because he can't fix the problem. In general, studies have shown that men tend to cope with the emotional stress of infertility by using denial, distancing, avoidance, and withdrawal, which may lead his partner to believe he is callous and disinterested.[25] . . . It is typical for the woman to want her husband to be more emotional and the husband to want his wife to be more rational. As a result, partners may begin to doubt the stability of the relationship and may withdraw from one another, feeling angry, hurt, and alone."[26]

Counseling can assist couples under these circumstances to develop more effective means of communication and a better understanding of each other's personal journey through infertility. The recipient father should be encouraged to explore what his dreams for his children might have been, and how he imagined his role as a father. He can be encouraged to explore how those dreams would be any different if he fathers a child whose genes he doesn't share.

On Using a Sperm Donor: Who's the Real Daddy?

If a man is feeling uncertain about his role because donor sperm is involved in making his family, he may find some clarity and solace in this wonderful article by Janet Falon that appeared in the Philadelphia Enquirer.

"On this Father's Day, my husband and I are trying to figure out who will be the father of our child. After five years of pain, invasive

---

[25] E. Grill, Psy.D., L. Josephs, Ph.D., and M. Brisman, J.D., "Assisted Reproduction," *Reproductive Medicine Secrets*, ed. P. Chan, MD, M. Goldstein, MD, and Z. Rosenwaks, MD (Philadelphia: Hanley & Belfus, Inc. 2004) 391.

[26] L. Applegarth, Ed.D. and E. Grill, Psy.D., "Psychological Issues in Reproductive Disorders," ibid. 342.

physical procedures and tens of thousands of dollars of high-tech interventions for infertility, Cary and I are attempting one last time to get me pregnant. We're far along in adopting a baby, too, but we're trying something new. This time, we're using a sperm donor. We're trying to pick the father of our child. It's like dating again, like answering personal ads—only kinkier, the closest Cary and I will ever come to swinging. We're looking for a third partner to join us in an extremely intimate experience. And as in a night of anonymous swinging, we'll never know the man's name.

"The sperm bank sent us an inventory of about 150 potential donors, each listed with the same information: Race, ethnicity (maternal and paternal), blood type, height, weight, eye color, hair color and type, skin tone, education (most advanced degree), occupation, interests and activities. Do we stick with something familiar, or do we expand our horizons? Should we pick a man with curly hair because that's how Cary's was before he started to lose it, or should we go with a redhead? Do we choose only a man with our religion, or with advanced degrees like ours because we hope these are somehow genetic—and do we pass by a man who lists gun-collecting, truck pulls, and Jerry Springer as his primary interests because we're afraid these preferences, too, might be genetic?

"We went through this a couple of years ago, when we used the first of two egg donors. We learned each woman's favorite color, food and car and whether she played sports or an instrument, and so much more.

"This time around feels different. With the egg donor, I knew that whatever child might develop would still grow in my body; I would be an active participant. I would feed it and shelter it until it was ready to debut in the world. It's like when I received sourdough-bread starter from a friend; the integral raw material came from someone else, but it was up to me to nurture it.

"Using a sperm donor feels different, I think, because Cary will be less present in the biology of things. This biological gap will be true for both of us if we end up bringing another heartbeat into our home by adoption. I know that even in a normal pregnancy, the man often feels less involved than the mother-to-be—but it's that man's genes that are developing into a tiny new person, and this won't be the case for us.

"But if there's one thing I've learned after 45 years of being a daughter, a man doesn't merit the title of capital-F "Father" just because his sperm has fertilized a woman's egg, and the process came to fruition nine months later. That's easy.

"To be a real father means active participation in growing a human being. It means doing, and caring, and being, and loving, behaviors I can—and do—count on Cary to perform. No matter what science was involved in creating the child, father isn't a noun—it's a verb. A very active verb."[27]

Mothers and Donor Sperm

The mother's issues concerning the use of donor sperm can be similar to the father's, even though her genetic and gestational continuity of parenthood are maintained. Like her husband, she too may feel that it's at least a little bit adulterous to accept into her body the life-giving cell of a male stranger. On the other hand, if she also recognizes that it is she and her husband who chose together the specific contribution to her ovum, the presence of a stranger's genes may not be such a problem. Again, counseling can be very helpful to couples sorting out the intimate presence of a stranger.

The wife in this situation can be enormously helpful to her husband as he grieves the loss of his genetic connection. She might want to acknowledge that it would have been wonderful to see some of those physical traits and talents she admires in him, but the traits she most admires in him are his values and beliefs, not his genes. Those values and beliefs, she can point out, will be what he transmits

---

[27] Janet Falon, *Philadelphia Enquirer*, 18 June 2000. Janet Ruth Falon is a writer and writing teacher in Elkins Park, PA. She has an essay in the book *Father: Famous Writers Celebrate the Bond Between Father and Child*, edited by Claudia O'Keefe (Pocket Books).

to their child through his nurturing, and she can stress that she looks forward to that special aspect of his participation.

Helpful counseling might include a discussion of how intimately a person's basic nature is affected by the nurturing environment in which he or she was raised. Once the loss of genetic connection is acknowledged and grieved, the recipient mother and father can move on to imagine how they would like to nurture their future child together.

Fathers and Donor Ovum

A father's issues with donor ovum usually involve helping his wife deal with her sense of lost genetic connection. As he dreamed of making a family with his wife, he surely felt drawn to special qualities that he hoped their children would inherit. When he discovers that this dream is not to be, he can feel deep personal disappointment, as well as a sense of loss for his wife. Accepting an ovum from another woman does not involve his having to take that ovum into his body, but that doesn't mean there aren't issues for him to work through.

In her work as an infertility counselor, Judith Kottick sees a wide range of feelings from recipient fathers of donor ova. "Some men are more devastated than their wives about the loss of her genetic contribution," she says. "Having sought out their wives and chosen them based on qualities they admire, they want those same qualities in a child. When another woman's ovum is necessary to conceive, they can be deeply distressed at what they believe their potential child may be missing out on. Some husbands can be even more selective about their donor than their wives—and more intent on finding the 'perfect match,' as they feel they have found in their wife. Other men, however, may find the donation of ovum easier to accept because their own genetic contribution remains intact. Their concern may center more around their wife's emotional reaction and how to make her feel comfortable . . . . It is definitely important for husband and wife to be respectful of each other's position, and this is not always easy. At a time when you need your spouse to be in sync more than ever, it can be extremely lonely and isolating to find that you are emotionally at odds. At times like this, I highly recommend counseling or support groups."[28]

Husbands and wives can provide immeasurable support to each other by reminding themselves that they have begun this journey together and have selected a donor for certain qualities they both admire. A husband will want his wife to know that, for him, making such a selection in no way replaces the special love he feels for her. He might find reassurance—and affirmation in the relationship—if he can acknowledge that it is a precious measure of her love for him that she is willing to accept whatever help they need so that they can raise a family together.

In my case, when the possibility of ovum donation was first suggested to us, David thought the entire idea was pretty bizarre, but after reflection, his feelings shifted. "At first, I wondered why would I want to conceive a child with anybody's egg beside Lonny's and perhaps miss some of those wonderful qualities I saw in our other children that were surely a part of her," he recalls. "She's vivacious, a bit crazy, willing to adventure into the unknown, has a highly developed sense of social justice, and can put the shyest patient at ease within minutes of meeting her. Most unnerving is her uncanny ability to sense what she feels the universe is asking of us, and to do whatever must be done to realize our dreams. However, having journeyed at her side through this wonderful world over these many years, and having experienced how often her intuition has been right on the mark, I found my initial reservations melting away and soon became infected with her enthusiasm to have a baby again."

In becoming a father again, David claims his most amazing discovery has been seeing in our youngest son, just as he has in our older children, qualities he'd once assumed would have been the product of my genes. "It's obvious that our son has a strong intuitive connection with his mother," he says. "Tucker captures her light in

---

[28] Author's personal correspondence with Judith Kottick.

his own mischievous smile, is passionate in expressing what he likes and dislikes, just like his mother, and shows his gentle reassuring nature to others when they need it, just like his mother does. Yes, he can tease and cajole when he wants to get his way, and he is quite the articulate negotiator, too—all traits Lonny says he gets from me—but it is clear to me that he is so much a part of us both that the idea he might have lost out on anything Lonny would have passed on genetically was set aside long ago."

Mothers and Donor Ovum

The mother who carries a baby created with the help of donor ovum faces unique concerns for which there has been no grounding experience within our society. No matter how comforted she feels that her husband's sperm helped start new life within her, she may feel, nevertheless, that she is carrying a little stranger.

For some women, a mother's feeling of being unrelated and disconnected may simply reflect a natural curiosity, a desire to get to know her child better. For others, it may indicate a mother's need to work through her understanding of maternal lineage in the context of her personal family history. In some instances, the need to "de-strange" the child can reflect a lack of confidence to trust in the natural, pre-programmed process of bonding because she pursued an "unnatural" process to become pregnant. It is very common for donor ovum recipients to fear that they will not be able to bond as intimately with this child in utero and after birth.

Paradoxically, the mother may also feel an unanticipated, yet strong bond with her donor. I had one patient who took this so far in her own mind that after her baby was born, some of her post-partum angst had to do with imagined worries about her donor. Would the donor regret her decision? Did she need reassurance that her gift was truly appreciated and cherished? Would she feel abandoned somehow? Fortunately, her husband was able to help her redirect her protective and maternal energy towards their family and restore the donor to her proper place in the entire scheme of things.

Considerations When Choosing a Donor

Here are some questions you might ask yourself as you consider sperm or ovum donation:

- Do I have clarity about my own identity, so that I can raise a child produced by ART to be a self-confident and healthy adult?
- Do I care whether the donor already has had children of his or her own? (Some recipient couples feel that a donor's having had children increases the likelihood that the donor's decision was mature and well informed.)
- Does the donor's religious or ethnic background matter?
- How important is donor appearance and/or intelligence?

Here are some questions to ask about the donor you are considering:

- Is there any family history of alcoholism, depression, mental illness, cancer, early onset heart disease, hypertension, diabetes, or birth defects?
- How many times has this donor already contributed? (Some argue that a limit of six should be set for ovum donations so that the donor's ovarian reserve is not threatened should she decide to expand her own family. A case can also be made for placing some reasonable limit on the number of donations a sperm bank should accept from a single donor. The use of sperm from a single donor to impregnate a large number of women in one geographic region creates a risk, albeit small, that offspring from the donor might one day meet and marry.)
- What were the pregnancy outcomes from previous attempts?
- Has an egg donor had any complications from prior stimulation?
- Are there any red flags in the donor's personal health history that might make him or her a poor candidate? (Is the donor a carrier

- for Tay Sachs disease, Cystic Fibrosis, or other equally serious inherited disorders that could be passed on to offspring?)
- Is there a history of alcohol or drug abuse? (Substance abuse is a red flag for emotional instability and a propensity to addictions that may be inherited.)
- Are there any health problems with the donor's children, such as behavioral problems, congenital birth defects, chronic illnesses, or developmental delays?
- Does the donor clearly understand the boundaries of the proposed arrangement and feel comfortable with them?

The Donor-Recipient Contract

Although most major programs have their own legal forms and don't require an outside contract, I recommend that you consult a lawyer to create a legal document spelling out all the details of your particular donor arrangement. I found that my clinic's contract was inadequate for all my considerations. Here's an overview of what such a contract might cover:

- All rights and responsibilities involving the use of ova or sperm following retrieval are transferred to the recipient couple.
- All responsibility for a child born of an ART pregnancy is that of the parent recipients, including provision for all medical, financial, and emotional care, regardless of special needs.
- Disposition of any unused embryos should be spelled out. What will be done with them a) when the parents have completed the family building for which the embryos were created, b) if the parents divorce, or c) if one parent dies or becomes permanently disabled? Options for disposition include: having the laboratory thaw them and return them to the parents for private burial; donating them to an infertile couple, donating them for scientific research, and cryopreserving them for possible life-saving cellular therapy (e.g., using them as a source of stem cells to treat a condition that a child might develop in the future).

The Confidentiality Questions:

Do You Want to Know your Donor?

In every ART experience that involves third party participation, the question arises: do you and your donor want to know each other? I have met donors who think of their gift as akin to an organ donation and have no need or desire to connect with the recipient couple or the child. Others would like the opportunity to get to know the recipient couple and to meet the child that results from their assistance.

That was how it was with my donor. My donor and I met even before my husband and I had decided we would go the egg donor route. She and I elected to stay in touch after the donation and have built a sister-like bond over the years that we've known each other. (Our children have also come to know each other, but more about this in Chapter 8, where I discuss how to tell children their own stories.)

As I've said, my case is unusual. In most instances, the relationship boundaries with anonymous donors are clearly defined by provider programs, and they usually require strict anonymity for parents as well as donors. In many cases, only non-identifying health history is available.

Some ovum donor resources do allow parents and donors to specify the degree of anonymity with which they are comfortable—for example, whether the parents would allow the clinic to let the donor know whether his or her contribution resulted in a live birth. In other instances, donors can indicate if they would be willing to allow a recipient child to contact them when the child reaches adulthood, or if they would be willing to write a letter for parents to share with their child when he/she is ready, describing why they decided to be a donor. Some agencies are willing to provide the parent with pictures and/or the opportunity to meet and interview the donor. Some donors are quite happy to have parents exchange occasional letters or holiday cards with them from time to time if that would give the parents comfort, but the decision about contact should be based on the parents' desires and the donor's receptivity—in that order.

I've heard some therapists ask: "What about the child? Isn't it up to the child to say what he or she prefers?"

I believe that such a line of thinking reflects poor judgment. It is not up to our children to choose for themselves whether or when they are ready to know identifying information about their parents' donors. ART parents are just as capable as any other parents of making such decisions on behalf of their children in a manner that honors their unique family values. As I've said before, all children have the right to feel, first and foremost, an exclusive connection to their primary family of origin. No one can know better than parents what should be disclosed to children about the circumstances of their conception, and when the disclosure should be made. The Ethics Committee of the American Society for Reproductive Medicine addresses this issue, encouraging parents to consider disclosure while recognizing that the decision is a personal one to be made by the parents themselves.[29] In Chapter 8, I discuss in some detail the issue of disclosure of birth origins to ART children, describing not only the experiences of ART parents who opted for disclosure, but also the experiences of ART children learning about their origins, told in their own words.

Should You be Open about Using ART?

Do you want the world to know your secret? Some parents fear that exposing the truth may jeopardize the future well being of their child. Many couples are also afraid of the reactions of others. Here are some stories that illustrate how some couples are facing the dilemma:

Bernadette: Still Undecided

"I gave birth to twins by ovum donation just a year ago. My husband and I still have not resolved whether/when to tell our babies

---

[29] Ethics Committee Report, "Informing Offspring of their Conception by Gamete Donation," *Fertility and Sterility* Vol. 81, No. 3, March 2004.

that they are not genetically related to me. Until we resolve that issue, we have kept the information private. Although I still struggle with when/whether/how to tell the babies, I must say that when viewing parenthood in its entirety, the issue of the embryo itself seems so small compared with all that is entailed in bringing a life into this world and nurturing that life after birth. The embryo itself, very precious, is only one part of all that parenthood encompasses, and all that you and your partner (if you have one) will have been through.

"Now that I have two toddlers and I have been through the pregnancy, bed-rest, childbirth, a premature delivery and neonatal unit experience, breastfeeding, napping, colic, etc., etc . . . . gee whiz, the issue of whose genetic material helped start their lives seems so infinitesimally small. I know that in the midst of the pregnancy it seems so very important—and it is, but there are many other important aspects/contributions to your baby's life. As time goes on, and your attachment, investment, and sacrifice for your baby increase, I think you'll find that the genetic material is no more important to your baby's life than all that you will contribute: healthy eating during pregnancy, cuddling and nuzzling the baby after birth, waking up every 3 hours round the clock to feed him/her, running out for diapers, having a family photo taken and for the first time not caring how your photo turns out because you are hoping your baby's shining personality is captured on film, comforting your baby during colic/indigestion/bad dreams, holding a freezing cold teething toy on her gums to provide relief during teething, etc. The issue of where we each come from cannot be ignored. Yet it is not the only thing, either."

Kendra: Single Mom

"Given our societal biases on so many things, will my child be at a disadvantage by being from donor ovum and donor sperm? What will others think of him and how will they treat him? Will they treat him differently than they would have had he been a natural child? Will they treat me differently? Will I care? These are rhetorical questions. But they are also issues I need to deal with as I go through the process of fully embracing my need for a donor embryo.

"When a child becomes a reality in my life, it is possible that I will want to share with others the miracle that brought him to me. Once 'told,' one cannot 'un-tell.' I don't know how these decisions will affect my life or the life of my child, and I feel it necessary to protect the privacy of both of us from the unknown.

"My situation is complicated by the fact that I am single. If I were part of a couple, it's very unlikely that I would give my child details about how she was conceived. Because I am single, I may need to provide more information than the norm. This is where the stigma aspect is raised. Would it be different if our society were more open minded and accepting of alternate parenting methods? Donor egg . . . donor sperm . . . donor embryo are all marvelous ways of achieving a biological (though not necessarily a genetic) family. But it is a complicated situation.

"Maybe by the time it matters, the outside world will be more understanding. I mean, who even thinks about Louise Brown, the first test tube baby. Will it be the same for genetic sharing one day? I hope so."

Irina: Religious and Ethnic Considerations

"I think openness is necessary, because your child's genetic origins are about her body and her identity, not yours.

"I am Jewish, and my egg donor comes from an Irish Catholic family. My husband is French and Protestant. For me to raise my child 100% Jewish Ashkenazi (family roots are in Russia), disregarding all else and not take into account her genetic roots from Ireland would be, for me, disrespectful to the child, just as much as raising my child without awareness of her lineage and cultural, religious history from France. For me, it's a matter of one's personal history. While I don't make a big deal of lineage, it is the nature of most people to be interested in their roots and ancestry, and it is dishonest to pass our (as DE recipients) genetic heritage off as belonging to the child. History is important; the knowledge of our roots has somehow shaped all of our lives.

"Yet, the facts of our child's genetic background, and her knowledge of it, doesn't make us any less their mothers. Our cultural, religious history is integral to our child's development. History is just that . . . . Parenting is the 'here and now,' and who is changing all those dirty diapers.

"Another angle to consider is about the 'here and now' fifteen years from now. Have you thought about if DNA 'finger printing' were to become a weekend science project that your kid brings home to test on mommy and daddy? She'll have a hard time understanding why mommy doesn't want to do a skin or nail scraping for the test.

"Each choice—to tell or not tell—is individual. However, I think that as we make our decision to tell or not to tell, we should ask ourselves all the reasons why we should or shouldn't tell. Whatever answer we come to from this internal dialogue, it should never be based on our own selfishness, trepidation, or shame. It should be based on what belongs to the child and what is in her/his interest to know."

Krista: Responding Creatively to Friends

"When I got 'Congratulations!' on my pregnancy, in person, I returned thanks and offered a few noncommittal, but sincere comments. I often said, simply 'My husband and I have struggled so long to be able to share a full-term pregnancy together. It's such an incredible bond. We feel so incredibly blessed!'"

Annabelle: Feeling Isolated by Secrecy

"I cannot tell any of my family members that my child is by ovum donation because they would shun him as unrelated. Although I work with wonderful people, I cannot tell any of my colleagues about my infertility or use of donor ovum because I think they would view me as a freak.

"I am very lucky that I have made a number of contacts with other women in my area who are going through the ovum donation process or already have children by ovum donation. These women are now my closest friends, because we share a unique bond. And, no matter how hard it is to answer those who ask where my son got his beautiful blue eyes (my husband and I both have brown eyes), I will always be thankful that the donor ovum option exists, that I took it, and that it worked for me."

Katerina: Protecting her Child's Privacy

"During my ovum donation, I told no one, and I held my husband to complete secrecy. I believe that it is the child's right to know before anyone else. So if you decide to tell your children when they are old enough, then they are the first to know—and only ones to know—if that is their wish.

"Just as people are always asking about our adopted Russian son's family in Russia, it will be up to our new baby to decide who should know his history.

"I think you have to be careful whom you tell, and why. I have seen families use the circumstance of donor ovum and donor sperm as a power play, to gain sympathy, as arguments in a divorce case, (she's not really the bio mother so the father should get custody or vice versa!), to assign blame for a child's behavior or personality traits, etc.—but most often by brothers—and sisters-in-law who are vying for 'more validity' for heirlooms, wills, etc.—and no matter how much you want to confide in someone you think you can trust, . . . people never keep their mouths shut. Your child ends up with no control over who knows everything about his origins—something he might have chosen to keep personal if he were given the chance."

Christina: Telling Only Those Who've Had the Experience

"It has been so interesting seeing the responses from our friends and family over the past months. At this point, I am very open about my struggles to get pregnant and the use of IVF. I am happy to answer questions, and I feel that I am helping others understand newer technology and what miracles are available now. However, when it comes to donor ovum, I tell only other infertile women whom I think I can help. I do plan on being open with my daughter about her genetic origins.

"One thing I do warn others about: Don't tell anyone unless you are prepared for others to find out. A friend of mine told only her parents and in-laws. Soon after, she was at a brunch with other family members when her uncle asked, loud and clear across the table, 'So, what did the donor look like?' She was in tears. This is the reality—people talk."

A Lesson of History—and Secrecy

During the 1950s, 60s and 70s, couples who underwent donor insemination due to male infertility were firmly advised never to tell anyone of their children's origins. Most of these children were raised to adulthood having no idea that a male donor played a role in their conception history.

Today, a number of these adults have finally been told or recently discovered their complete genetic origins. A number of them refer to themselves now as "DI adoptees" (donor insemination adoptees). They feel deprived of an important part of their identity in not knowing the man who donated half of the blueprint for their chromosomes, and they are spending a considerable amount of time and effort in searching for their "genetic fathers."

The fact that these adults call themselves DI adoptees deeply saddens me because the term "adoptee" glosses over important distinctions between adoption and the ART experience. First of all, children created from donor sperm were not pre-existing beings, adopted by a family different from their birth parents. Second, their self-designation as adoptees ignores their mother's genetic and gestational role in their creation. And third, they disenfranchise the fathers whose dreams, shared and pursued with their wives, of becoming parents are the basis for their existence in the first place.

Can anyone be half-adopted? Is there really a genetic father out there who gave up half a baby for adoption? It doesn't make sense. What does make sense is to acknowledge and honor the fact that there is a male donor who gave this child's parents a life-giving cell that helped them to create him. No one questions that this is a valuable contribution, and most would agree that the child deserves to know that the donor's cell may carry with it important medical history. And many people believe that the child has a right to know about, and even to seek out, the donor to learn more about his genetic background. I have no argument with these views. But this is a far cry from trying to attach the notion of parent to a donor who never laid eyes on his offspring, who never had the desire to create him, and who invested none of the love and commitment that all ART couples invest in order to become parents.

Messages to Give Yourself

It takes multiple tools to make it through the ART experience. One device that has worked for me is to remember the following statements, even repeat them to myself in times of stress:

- Of course, I feel insecure sometimes.
- Before this success, I endured many failures.
- All parents, no matter how they become parents, need nurturing and reassurance.
- My issues now may not be my children's issues in the future.
- The only reason our children exist is because of the paths we have taken to bring them to life.
- We deserve each other. We're a family!

For Mothers:

- Receiving an embryo created by another into my body may feel like I'm accepting a little stranger, but the biological mothering I give to him now is just the beginning of a long, rewarding and intimate relationship.

For Fathers:

- Being a father means active participation in growing a human being. It means doing, and caring, and being, and loving. No matter what science was involved in creating my child, "father isn't a noun—it's a verb. A very active verb."[30]

---

[30] Falon.

Chapter 5

The Surrogate Experience

Surrogacy is a special kind of donor assistance that deserves its own chapter for a number of reasons. For one, the surrogate is a woman who sustains new life by providing her uterus and body to grow and give birth to a baby—and that is a very big, very intimate involvement. For another, there are two types of surrogacy available: traditional and gestational. Each one presents unique issues for families to consider carefully.

Despite what you might think based on a few cases that made big headlines years ago, surrogacy actually goes smoothly most of the time. It does, however, necessitate a lot of thought and preparation. Some facts:

The *traditional surrogate* can become pregnant in two ways: either by intrauterine insemination with the expectant father's sperm, or by ovarian stimulation with fertility drugs to harvest her eggs, which are then fertilized in the lab with the intended father's (or donor's) sperm and transferred back to her uterus. In either scenario, the traditional surrogate's own eggs are used, and she carries the growing child for the intended parents. This form of surrogacy is less commonly used today since IVF and other ART options became available in the mid 1980's, making it possible to successfully transfer to the mother embryos created with a donor ovum and the expectant father's sperm. Traditional surrogacy is legal now only in certain states.

Traditional surrogacy arrangements can be emotionally complex. If the surrogate has other children, they may wonder why their mother would give away a baby who is related to them. The surrogate's partner also may have misgivings about his wife receiving and carrying another man's sperm. In light of this, professional surrogacy organizations should not only offer background checks and comprehensive counseling for all surrogate candidates, they should also interview the surrogate's husband or partner to explore his feelings about the intended arrangement.

The second surrogacy option is *gestational surrogacy*, in which a growing embryo belonging to the intended parents, and usually genetically related to both intended parents, is transferred to a designated carrier. The gestational carrier shares no genes with the child she bears, so it is less likely that she or her family will develop proprietary feelings for the child. Even so, she is likely to form an intimate, if short-term, emotional connection to the child during gestation.

A surrogacy organization must carefully identify and coordinate the expectations of all the participants. Numerous financial and contractual issues must be addressed. An experienced reproductive law specialist will also be needed to assist with establishing legal parental status by whatever means may be required. In some states, the couple that has provided the embryo to the gestational carrier may not be recognized as the child's legal parents without an order of the probate court that can only be obtained after the child's birth. Absent such an order, the assignment of post-delivery rights and responsibilities in a surrogacy contract may not be given effect should a dispute arise between parents and surrogate. And in some states, surrogacy arrangements in general, or certain provisions in surrogacy contracts, might be viewed by the courts as void or voidable at the option of the surrogate.

For these reasons, it is very important to consult an attorney about the surrogacy laws in the state where you live *and* in the state where your intended surrogate lives to be sure that all provisions in the contract you and your surrogate sign will be recognized and enforced by the courts in such states. There are now a number of law practices that specialize in infertility/reproductive law to assist intended parents with surrogacy arrangements.

Appropriate professional psychological counseling is also essential for all parties involved in surrogacy prior to a baby's conception. Careful discussions are needed about any on-going relationship between the parents and later the child, on the one hand, and the gestational carrier and her family on the other. Many recipient families choose to maintain contact with their surrogate after their baby is born, but if they make this choice, they should work with the help of a counselor to establish whatever relationship boundaries may be necessary very early on.

Above all, the assistance of a professional counselor is needed, both during the nine months of the pregnancy and beyond, to help the parents understand and cope with inevitable emotions surrounding the relinquishing of the mother's role in the direct nurturing of their baby during the pre-natal period. Giving birth represents one of the primal passages of life, and when it is entrusted to a third party, it can be deeply missed.

"For many women, giving up the pregnancy experience is *huge*," says Judith Kottick. "It speaks to the core of a woman's identity. I have heard patients say that they feel they are letting their child down even before they are born, because they are unable to nourish their baby in the womb."

It can be extremely difficult for a woman to watch someone else carry her baby effortlessly, especially if she has chosen surrogacy after multiple miscarriages. She can feel eternal gratitude to the carrier and resentment at the same time.

"Unlike egg donation, where there may be very little or no contact with the donor, with surrogacy, the more contact, the better," Kottick goes on to explain. "Most of these arrangements work out amazingly well, but when there are problems, they can be really ugly!! The stakes are high, and the emotions are so primitive and powerful. In the end, the carrier has so much power—no one can make her do anything with her body that she doesn't want to do. This is why I encourage intended parents to create the best relationship possible with their carriers. It is understood among professionals in this field that the more the carrier bonds with the intended parents, the less likely she will bond with the baby, and the more incentive she will have to be receptive to and carry out the intended parents' wishes."[31]

Selecting a Surrogate

Surrogates are generally found two ways: through a surrogacy organization, or through the parents' own personal network of family and friends. A surrogacy organization offers the benefits of proper medical and psychological screening. If you are making private arrangements, your REI specialist should arrange for your surrogate to have complete medical screening and psychological evaluation.

Before you proceed, you and your doctor should have satisfactory answers to these questions:

- What is the surrogate's gestational history? Has she had any previous pregnancies? Any complications?
- Does she have any other health problems?
- Does she have access to quality prenatal care, and does her hospital have an NICU (neonatal intensive care nursery)?
- Has she successfully given birth before?
- Are her children living with her? How is their health?
- Is she in a stable home, not planning to move, and not on any governmental assistance?
- Would she be willing to carry a multiple pregnancy—triplets or more—for you?
- Would she be willing, in the case of multiples beyond twins, to participate in fetal reduction if the procedure were medically recommended for the sake of her health or the health of the surviving one or two fetuses?

---

[31] Author's personal correspondence with Judith Kottick.

- Would she be willing to terminate the pregnancy if a serious birth anomaly were discovered?
- How does she plan to communicate with her husband, children, and other family members about her surrogate pregnancy and delivery?
- Are her family and friends supportive of her decision?
- Have you agreed on who should attend the delivery? Has her request to have you present been approved by her doctor?
- Has the labor and delivery unit also been notified that you are the parents and are to be treated as such?
- If she currently has a partner, how does the partner feel about the pending arrangements?
- Has she had any episodes of post partum blues or depression?
- What kinds of boundaries need to be honored should your surrogate live near-by or be a member of your family and therefore likely to have an ongoing relationship with your child?
- How extensively will you be in communication with each other throughout the pregnancy?
- What plans would you like to have in place, regarding notification and participation once labor has begun?
- Would she agree to let you and partner be present in the operating room should a Caesarean delivery become necessary?
- What plans do you have for your post partum time together in hospital?
- Have you familiarized yourselves with the family laws of the state in which you plan your delivery? Does your surrogate understand them also?
- Have you formally settled all the legal issues between you?
- Are you willing to accept your surrogate's right to make independent decisions regarding her prenatal and delivery care?
- Is the surrogate willing to abide by any special requests that you might have, e.g., no smoking, alcohol, bleaching hair, etc.

A Tale of Two Surrogates

When you undertake to build your family in a partnership with another person, you understand that you are going to face risks. No matter how carefully you choose your surrogate and draw up your agreement, the journey may be, like so much that happens in life, vastly different from what you dreamed.

Take, for example, the story of Cynthia's first experience with surrogacy. She had five children from her first marriage, and she wanted to share parenthood again with her second husband, who had never had a child of his own. She became pregnant very quickly, but the daughter she carried was stillborn at term. Two years later, she miscarried again. She then considered both ovum donation and surrogacy. Given her medical history, she chose surrogacy—and then began a nine-month-long series of encounters with unhappy surprises.

"Our surrogate was from out of state," Cynthia recalls, "which was the first problem that created a number of stresses. But the biggest issue was primarily that she didn't communicate with us, kept us uninformed during most of the pregnancy, and refused to live up to our agreement. She didn't have any of the pre-natal care—blood-work, tests, etc.—that she'd said she would, and we were afraid to try to force her to comply. We were given only brief pre-natal reports when she felt like giving them to us. She did have an ultrasound because there was some bleeding, and her midwife sent her in. We were sent one ultrasound picture, but we didn't receive it until a month after it was taken, and I think we got it only because we sent her the money to pay for the procedure.

"In the end, she did not even tell us she'd gone into labor. She left a message saying the baby was here and we needed to come down and bring the balance of the fee. We didn't get to be at the delivery; our son was sixteen hours old when we first saw him.

"Then, after the fee was paid, the surrogate refused to sign the necessary papers to add my husband's name to the birth certificate. It took us eighteen months and another six hundred dollars to get her signature. By then we'd learned our lesson. Because of her unreliability, we knew we had to get all our paperwork completed before giving her that final payment. At that point, we also had her sign the papers I needed for a step parent adoption and to have an amended birth certificate completed with both my name and my husband's.

"We have no argument, though, with how things turned out. Our child is two years and seven months old now, and he's an absolute joy to us. The surrogate gave us a priceless, wonderful gift; she just did it in a horrible way."

Cynthia and her husband are now expecting another baby. This time, their experience with surrogacy is very different.

"Our second surrogate is from the same state where we live and where there are surrogate-friendly laws to support us," Cynthia says, "and that's changed everything. Our surrogate is a sweetheart, too. She is thirty-one and a mother herself of five children. She attends college and is an emergency medical technician. She says it is up to us how much contact we would want to have, and that is what we stated in our contract together. We have been visiting her from time to time during the pregnancy and staying in touch regularly through calls and email.

"With surrogacy, regardless of the contract, I truly believe you just have to trust each other and hope that everything will work out. It is important to try and find a surrogate who is mature and stable. Ideally, her focus should be based on the family she is helping. We have been truly blessed in finding our second surrogate."

My view on this situation is a little different. I believe it is in the best interest of everyone involved that the parties specify beforehand, by contract, that certain prenatal data will be shared in a timely manner by the surrogate's obstetrician with the parents in waiting. A signed release of medical information form should be filled out at the time of the contract and sent to the surrogate's obstetrician specifying what information needs to be copied and forwarded. Copies of a confirmed positive pregnancy test, blood type, expected date of delivery, and copies of serial ultrasound results, are examples of data that are important to have forwarded to the parents as pregnancy proceeds. Without this kind of information sent directly by the surrogate's obstetrician to the parents, there is no way for parents to confirm that a surrogate is actually pregnant and receiving the care for which they are paying.

The Womb Connection

How great is a woman's emotional attachment to her uterus? As the recent experience of my colleague, Sarah, illustrates, it can be as poignant and powerful as life itself.

At 35 years old, never married and childless, Sarah was diagnosed with an invasive adenocarcinoma (cancerous lesion) of the cervix. Her gyn-oncologist advised her that she'd need a radical hysterectomy. But the findings on her diagnostic biopsy indicated that the lesion, though extensive on the surface, had not progressed deeply into the cervical wall, and Sarah wondered if it might be possible to save her uterus through a new procedure called a radical trachelectomy (removal of most of the cervix, adjacent tissue, and pelvic lymph nodes, but leaving behind the uterus, tubes, and ovaries).

The problem was that her surgeon in New York had performed only 22 of these procedures and seemed to dismiss the urgency of her questions that centered on saving her uterus. Her parents, too, were concerned about her focus on saving her uterus when her life was at stake.

In exploring her feelings with me, Sarah was frank. "I honestly don't believe losing my life is the biggest issue for me right now. I feel I can beat this cancer. What is hardest for me is the feeling of castration I have about losing my uterus." Sarah felt deeply connected to the dream that one day she would bring new life into her world with a beloved partner. "This dream gives me something to live for," she said.

We discussed how important it was that Sarah be her own advocate—and how the choices she made in her own best interests for her body and spirit were as important to her eventual recovery as anything that could be done for her surgically.

Sarah consulted a reproductive specialist who reviewed with her how her eggs and/or ovaries could be saved, in case she needed radiotherapy following her operation. Then she and I carefully envisioned each possible future scenario. I explained that if it turned out that she would have to lose her uterus, there are wonderful women in this world who serve as gestational carriers, one of whom we would surely find to carry her baby for her, one day.

After considering all her options, Sarah made the brave decision to travel to Canada where Dr. Marie Plante and her associate had already performed over 85 radical trachelectomies, continuing the pioneering surgery originally developed by the French surgeon, Dr. Daniel Dargent.[32] As of this writing, we're waiting to see if there will be need for further treatment, but Sarah's preliminary results look hopeful.

It is just as devastating for some women to lose the intimate connection to pregnancy as it is for others to lose the intimate connection to genetic lineage—no single aspect of having children is more important than another. All women who need the reproductive assistance of another woman and turn to a traditional surrogate or gestational carrier act with great faith and courage. They journey further than any spontaneous parent could imagine and, as a consequence, become some of the finest parents a child could ever hope to have.

---

[32] According to Dr. Plante, after ten years of experience, the radical trachelectomy appears to be a valuable option for young women who wish to preserve their fertility potential. The oncologic and obstetrical results are encouraging. The recurrence rate for cancer cells following radical trachelectomy is comparable to the recurrence rate following a standard radical hysterectomy for the same size lesions. In Dr. Plante's practice, there have been 50 pregnancies from 31 of her patients; 75% of those pregnancies reached term, and all the deliveries were by C-section. Author's private correspondence with Dr. Plante.

What is a Parent? A Global Perspective

ART with third party assistance raises, and will continue to raise, a host of questions regarding what, exactly, is a parent. Before ART became available, it was pretty much assumed in Western culture that the genetic, gestational, and nurturing aspects of parenthood came as a complete package within one and the same person whom we refer to as the "parent." But as you sort out these questions for yourself and face the social, legal, and personal implications of being an ART parent needing gamete or carrier assistance, it might help to take a world view.

During the seven years that I spent traveling and working in the Pacific, it became clear to me that these island cultures had much more to say to me about parenting than did my own culture. They clearly helped evolve my concept of parenting as a role derived primarily from the intention to raise a child. In Micronesia and Polynesia, for example, the concept of parenthood is linked first and foremost to the commitment to love and nurture, and is not necessarily linked to any genetic or biological relationship. In the Marshall Islands, children are very often raised by aunts or uncles rather than their genetic parents. There isn't even a word in the Marshallese language for "cousin." To a Marshallese child, her cousins who are raised in her household are all her brothers and sisters.

In Hawaii, "aunty" and "uncle" are terms used not only for blood relations, but also for those elders who are respected and valued for the guidance they offer. In Hawaii, many children are raised by their grandparents when parents cannot manage the responsibilities of child rearing. These grandparents are often referred to as the child's "hanai" parents. "Hanai" literally means "to nurture." Historically, a traditional Hawaiian family would "hanai out," or give away, their first-born son to his paternal grandparents, or their first-born daughter to her maternal grandparents, to be raised. These children regarded their grandparents as their "hanai" parents, but they also maintained a close relationship with their birth parents. One important purpose of this historical practice was to ensure that the lore and special skills of the family would be passed on from generation to generation.

This was not the only instance in which a child would be "hanai'd out." Often, if a man and woman were found to be barren, a child would be given as a gift or blessing to this couple to raise, sometimes by someone completely unrelated. Even today in Hawaii, this tradition continues.

Western society needs to re-examine assumptions about what it is to be a parent. Sadly, we have a long way to go. Look, for example, at all the value-laden modifiers we have in the English language related to the concept of being a parent. We refer to "step parents," "foster parents," "adoptive parents," "genetic parents," "birth parents," "biological parents," "real parents," "true parents," "natural parents," and "surrogate parents," just to name a few. True, these terms are sometimes helpful in drawing distinctions for some legitimate purpose, but they are too often used to diminish somehow the status of a couple that is forced to turn to ART to realize the dream of loving, nurturing, and raising a child of its own.

Bearing Her Sister's Baby

Very often the kind of woman who offers to help another couple through surrogacy is someone who has had positive prior pregnancy experiences and enjoys the physiologic changes attending pregnancy. She is usually someone of high self-esteem who wants to be able to give someone else the same joy of raising children that she herself has experienced. Here's Jan's story:

"I am so thrilled that the twins I carried for my sister are finally with their mother and father. It was so heartwarming to see how happy my sister was at last, holding and loving those two precious little angels. I got to spend time with them in the hospital while I was recovering from the birth. Once all of us were released, I got to spend five days with my sister and her baby boys before they left. It was wonderful.

"Still, it was a lot harder than I expected, seeing them all get on that plane to head home. The tears were flowing freely, but seeing how happy my sister was at last, made it all worthwhile. We waited so long and finally the happy days are here.

"My own two children, Kenny, seven, and Sabrina, six, were wonderful while their cousins were here, grinning from ear to ear and wanting to hold them, but still fully understanding that the babies would not be staying. Kenny has been so sweet—he gives me extra hugs and kisses, saying, 'That's to make you happy since you are sad that Aunty's babies are gone.' I am doing fine, but I sure would love it if they lived closer so I could see them more often. Sabrina was just amazed that the babies were so small, but she kept saying, 'They are so pretty, Mom. Aunty must be so happy they are here.' I really do think both children are proud of me and of the whole process.

"I talk daily with my sister, and she tells me how the babies are doing and any cute things they have done. I am pumping my breasts and shipping the milk to her so the twins will have the best, healthiest start possible. My heart is so full of love for my sister, as well as for her beautiful boys, and I am so proud to have been able to bring them all together at last.

"Seeing the boys in my little sister's arms, my heart was just about bursting with joy, at last to be able to see her experiencing the wonder of motherhood. I can so easily go back to how overjoyed I was when I held each of my babies for the first time and how happy I still am each and every time I see, hold, or simply think of my own son and daughter and how they have enriched our lives."

No Greater Gift

I believe the world is a better place for the energy and the spirit of giving that surrogate mothers display. I am thankful that there are women willing to take such a pioneering journey, who give new meaning to the boundaries of love, female bonds, and the creation of a family.

Jackie, who has helped three couples become parents through a private arrangement and through the British organization, Childlessness Overcome Through Surrogacy (COTS), shares her story:

"I had four children, two boys and two girls, but I still had the need to do something else with my life. I began to investigate surrogacy after reading an article about it in a women's magazine. My children are the world to me. I try to imagine the pain if I had not been able to have them, and I don't think I could have coped. To me, the love for a child is bigger than everything else.

"At first, becoming a surrogate was a wild idea. I never thought it would happen. But then I met a couple; they weren't what I'd imagined they'd be like, but I saw that I could help them. So I was inseminated with the intended father's sperm. I was really pleased when I became pregnant right away. At three months, I was troubled by the idea that I would be betraying the baby inside of me by giving it away—it had total faith in me. But I think the hormones were working on my body and mind, making it hard for me to cope. And I never considered changing my mind. I never forgot that the baby was not mine but had been created because this couple was desperate to have a child. I could never go back on a decision of such huge importance. I trusted the couple to love the baby—as they trusted me to carry it and then say good-bye. They were with me when I gave birth to their 9lbs. 7oz. boy.

"The following weeks were really hard. My breasts filled with milk, and I would wake in the night and remember the baby was gone. It was grieving, but again I think hormones played a big part. I knew I was responsible for the baby's birth, but I didn't think of him as mine.

"I had two more babies with the same method for a lovely couple. The wife was born without a womb, so her only hope to have a family was through someone like me. We became good friends, and both parents were present at the births of the boy and the girl that I carried and delivered for them. The experiences we shared created a strong bond between us, not like a regular friendship. We have a special place in each other's hearts that I think will remain forever.

"I've heard it said that it is easier to be a gestational carrier—to just carry the genetic child of the couple—so this led me to try a 'host' pregnancy. It took three implantation attempts for me to get pregnant. I spent over a year trying to make the dream of a baby come true for another wonderful couple.

"Last June, I had their baby girl. (I can now say that both forms of surrogacy felt the same.) Now, I hear from the mum every day. She calls me her angel and tells me that she can still find herself standing with tears flowing down her face whenever she looks at her beautiful daughter, whom she thought she might never have.

"Surrogacy is not an easy thing to do. It can take over your life. But once you have shared such an experience, it is hard to stop. I wish I could help everyone, but I know that, at age 38, my days of being a surrogate are coming to an end. It has been a wonderful experience, and I have gained a great deal from meeting some very brave couples."

Chapter 6

Pregnant at Last!

In 1995, when I made my personal entry into the world of ART, I struggled with my decision and all the ramifications of it without the counseling that I surely could have used. There I was, a fully informed Ob/Gyn, with all the advantages of knowing what medical science could offer, yet I was just as susceptible as any other woman to the emotional consequences of navigating those uncharted waters.

Prior to my ART pregnancy, I was given a single psychological phone interview by a nurse/social worker, for which I was charged $200. Her questions centered on our family but were limited to whether my husband was supportive of my desire, why at my age I wanted to have more children, etc. The questions were not geared to elicit any deep emotional material, and there was absolutely no exploration of the issues that might come up later for me or for my family.

In the beginning, I wrestled with whether I had the right to avail myself of the advantages of ART. I already had two healthy children. Should I be taking up a clinic's time and space as a patient? Perhaps I should just be out there educating infertile couples and getting them into the system in my place? The idea of adoption as an alternative to ART raised similar feelings for me. Families who might never otherwise know the joy of rearing children should come first, I reasoned. Though I would have loved to adopt a child, I felt, in doing so, I might be taking a precious opportunity away from another deserving couple. At the onset of my journey, these doubts needed to be brought to light and resolved, and in retrospect I know that counseling would have helped me deal with them. But, alas, it was my experience to have to go it alone.

My Story: Facing the Unexpected

With my third pregnancy, there also came an onslaught of unanticipated worries and guilt. Whenever someone congratulated me, I felt a gnawing discomfort at not being completely forthcoming with every detail about how I'd achieved this miracle state, although I don't recall having any such guilt about not providing details of my other two children's conception and gestation. I was soon to discover I would be confronted with an entirely new host of emotional and physical challenges, unique to the timing and circumstances of this pregnancy.

In the weeks after the successful transfer of six embryos into my body, I was full of hope, and of anxiety. Returning to Hawaii, David and I stopped in Berkeley to spend the Thanksgiving holiday with our closest friends from college, Mary and Jason. They were all smiles, thrilled to hear everything about the miraculous medical journey David and I had embarked upon. But looking at them across the table, I kept remembering the terrible tragedy they'd faced twenty years earlier, with the loss of their only daughter. Not yet a year old, she was in her mother's arms having just finished breast-feeding, when she suddenly stopped breathing and turned a dusky blue. In spite of her mother's valiant efforts at CPR, an ambulance ride to Massachusetts General Hospital, and emergency cardiac surgery to try to stabilize her circulation, she died in the operating room. Mary and Jason were later to learn that their little girl had a silent blood vessel anomaly that deprived her of oxygen to her heart. My recollection chilled me to the bone. Here, with my pregnancy, was a time for peace and thankfulness, yet all I could think about was the unfairness of life and how my baby or babies might share a similar fate.

In mid-December, when I was five weeks pregnant, we flew to Utah to spend Christmas with medical friends from my residency days. Our two families were out on the slopes enjoying some deep powder while I waited at the foot of the mountain for them to join me for lunch in a little eatery called the Cookie Corner, filled with wonderful aromas. I was carrying what could be as many as six little embryos inside, but, oddly enough, at this time I wasn't worried.

Then suddenly, with no warning, I felt a painless gush of blood. "Oh my God, it's the babies!" I was thinking as I walked towards the restroom. I sat still and silent in the stall and watched as deep red clots of blood emerged from me. I could hear women coming and going in their clunky ski boots. I tried to remain calm. "Okay, there is no cramping; it may not be a miscarriage," I told myself. My uterus had not yet pushed out the embryos.

So, with determination and no inhibition whatsoever, I emerged from the stall with wads of toilet paper stuffed between my legs under my two layers of long underwear and walked carefully to the nearest lounge area where I proceeded to stretch out flat on the floor, oblivious to the public. "I am going to wait this out. I am going to take control of this," I thought. And there I remained, with the occasional curious onlooker asking me if I were all right as he or she carried a lunch tray to one of the nearby tables. I nodded to them, but my mind was a million miles away focused only on life in my womb. "Hold on," I mentally whispered to my babies. "Whoever must go, it is safe to leave, but if you are alive, just hold on. Mother is waiting for you. You can make it, little one."

Eventually my family arrived on the scene. I don't remember how they found me; it is all a blur. Somehow, they gently moved me back to our friends' home, and I remained on my back all the way, telling my womb to stay quiet and relaxed, not to cramp, no matter how much blood was coming out.

By morning, my bleeding had slowed to a trickle. My friend, who was also a physician, arranged for me to have an emergency ultrasound at the hospital. So we made our way into Salt Lake City. Although my blood loss had been substantial, I remained eerily serene. Just before the ultrasound was to begin, I announced that I knew I was still pregnant. I told the sonographer that although embryos were likely to have left my body, there hadn't been any definite sign of a miscarriage. He must have thought I was daft, considering how much blood I'd lost. But I knew, as sure as anything, that there was life still inside of me and that I wasn't in denial.

Sure enough, a few moments later, there before us on the screen, was a single pulsating point of life. My husband looked on in disbelief. And I was confirmed in my motherhood.

In February, at sixteen weeks along, I flew from Hawaii to Chicago to one of the country's most qualified specialists to perform my amniocentesis. Some might wonder why I would risk this precious baby by inserting a needle into its safe sanctuary. After all, the donor was still in her twenties, so a genetic amniocentesis wasn't warranted on the basis of advanced maternal age. But I had good reasons for going ahead with the test. As a mother nearly fifty years old, if I were to have a baby with a major problem, I knew that I might not be alive to care for the child through its adult years, not in the same way I would have with my older children had one of them been born with major medical problems. When I gave birth this time, complications would come with an entirely different set of consequences for my family. This responsibility was David's and mine, and as much as possible, we needed to be sure that there would be no surprises.

During the procedure, I waited to feel the tiny popping sensation as the needle penetrated the womb's wall. I told my baby to stay well away from that needle. The fluid came through clear, with no sign of bleeding or any cascading droplets into the womb's chamber. Then came the waiting to confirm what appeared to be an entirely healthy boy. Two weeks later, I was told, indeed, all was normal. Until then, I hadn't totally trusted that everything would work out.

My Story: Further Complications

The physical demands of this third pregnancy were not a problem for me, except that the early hemorrhaging had put me on bed rest for a few weeks, and I gained about forty pounds overall, instead of twenty-five as I had with each of my first two babies. I was active almost the whole time, swimming and walking, even working out with a trainer. Once I entered the last three months of my pregnancy (third trimester), however, my emotional and physical journey started to converge in a way I had not anticipated, my body forecasting where my mind was going.

Interrupted sleep had been normal for me for over twenty years. It wasn't unusual for me to be up throughout the night with a patient in labor, then make my 6:30 am rounds, grab a quick bite to eat in the hospital cafeteria, and be off to see my office patients throughout the day before returning home to my family. On any given night, I could be awakened and called to the emergency room. This was normal. The hallmark of my functioning in obstetrics was my ability to catch a few winks at the drop of a hat, in an empty room or on a couch in the doctors' lounge, and awaken refreshed on less than an hour or two of rest. But during my last two months of pregnancy, things changed.

Until about thirty-two weeks along, I was still able to handle my on-call schedule without difficulty, but I mentioned to my doctor that I was now experiencing air hunger at night and needed to yawn a lot to catch my breath. I also found that my legs were restless and jumpy whenever I lay down, and I would ask my husband to massage my calves to help me fall asleep. While he worked on one side, the other leg would tap, tap, tap against the bed sheet of its own accord, as if discharging some excess electrical current. I hardly slept at all. I just cat-napped during the nights.

My prenatal exams continued to show that I was in excellent health, so my doctor and I attributed my symptoms to the usual discomfort of an enlarging uterus pressing against the diaphragm and making breathing more difficult.[33] We missed the true diagnosis. My symptoms were the early signs of a deep anxiety, and at five weeks postpartum, without warning, they returned in a full-blown depression (more about this in Chapter 7).

---

[33] The diaphragm is a large muscle separating the abdominal cavity from the lungs. When the enlarging uterus takes up more and more space within the abdominal cavity, the diaphragm gets pushed upwards, leaving less room for the lungs to fully expand with inhalation. As a result, a sense of breathlessness can be experienced.

The Legacy of Infertility

Every first-time pregnant woman, no matter what her circumstances, experiences unexpected emotions. So it comes as no surprise that when a pregnancy is achieved through ART, after a long struggle filled with doubts and frustrations, emotional issues are not suddenly going to cease when mom gets pregnant. In most cases, dark, troubling feelings are going to continue to surface for the duration of the pregnancy and beyond. Some of the emotions can stem, as mine did, from a sense of undeserved privilege at availing oneself of the miracles of medical science when there are so many children in need of adoption. Others can come from the legacy of infertility and/or earlier traumatic experiences. All of these psychological issues need to be sorted out, processed, and let go, ideally with the help of a counselor.

Do you recall the picture of a happy mother holding her baby in her arms on the box of Ivory Snow detergent? For years, that image epitomized for me what becoming a mother would feel like, capturing the promise of a perfect outcome, with no room for fears, worries, or what-ifs. But if there is one thing that characterizes pregnancy after infertility, it is the distinct absence of the Ivory Snow mother's bliss! Many women who have endured years of infertility can't quite believe it when they have achieved a viable pregnancy. There is no way that they can ever return to the innocence of assuming that everything from here on will go smoothly. Nothing about the journey that brought them to this wondrous moment involved events that were going just right. Thus, in spite of the miracle at hand, their emotions may at times surprise and frighten them.

In the chat room of the online support group Mothers Via Egg Donation (MVED-L),[34] Renee, an expectant mother, chronicles her emotional turbulence this way:

---

[34] The American Surrogacy Center (TASC) at www.surrogacy.com provides comprehensive health and infertility-related support and information through various support groups, including MVED-L.

"I am grateful out of my mind to be pregnant. But a few things have happened this week that really surprised me. My friends now tell me about everyone they know who is pregnant or who just had a baby, assuming that because I am now expecting, I can relate.

"Well, I am shocked to realize I still can't relate to the experience of anyone who gets pregnant with tender lovemaking, or—worse—one friend who is expecting her 'oops!' fourth baby. I feel angry when anyone tries to compare our realities. The bottom line is: I'm furious at how unfair our struggle has been compared to that of other couples.

"I used to ride my bicycle everywhere. I rode it to work. It made me feel young and competent. But now my obstetrician doesn't think it's worth the risk for me to ride while I'm pregnant. And I agree. But this week at work, I was told about another colleague who rode her bike right up until her labor started!

"I am angry that I don't get to be a normal pregnant woman. I am jealous of women who don't worry, who assume everything will work out, and it does.

"I feel like all that innocence has been taken away from me. I am angry at how unfair all this has been: the money we've spent, the time I've lost being depressed, the friendships that have gone by the wayside, the way my life has fallen out of step with others my age, the feeling that creeps in when my husband and I make love—that I am an infertile woman.

"So I guess I'm sad that all these emotions are still with me, even though I am now pregnant. The feelings scare me because I don't want to be an angry woman for the rest of my life, and I don't want this baby to feel unwelcome because I didn't get to have a 'normal' pregnancy. I wonder if there are other women out there who have felt the same?"

The answer to Renee's question is an unequivocal "yes" from many women in the support group.

In my view, it takes integrity to look at anger, and it is the start of the process of healing and growth. Have you ever heard the she-wolf howl? Have you ever seen the rage of a mother bear? An infertile woman—who is also, of course, so much more—may join them. She is intimately within nature's path, not an angry woman for the rest of her life, but a woman who can embrace anger for what it is and move forward, to empower what she is becoming.

Michele is another expectant mother who, with all that she went through to become pregnant, still can't relax. She clearly expresses this ongoing anxiety when she pours out her heart with these concerns:

"I'm seventeen weeks pregnant via donor egg," she writes online, "and I'm wondering if those of you who have had a child worried that something would happen throughout your pregnancy. My husband and I tried to conceive for six years, and I've had two miscarriages. I thought that once I got pregnant and made it past twelve weeks, I could actually start enjoying the pregnancy . . . but I can't seem to let go of these irrational fears that something is going to happen. I started feeling movement two weeks ago. Now, if I don't feel fetal movement every day, I worry (although I know that at the beginning feeling the baby can be sporadic). I've also had spotting from a retained blood clot. Sometimes this has happened after intercourse, so now I'm afraid to have sex, even though the doctor says it's okay. This is wearing me down. Is it normal to worry like this?"

Several members of MVED-L are quick to respond.

"YES, YES, YES," Jennifer reassures Michele. "Your worries are absolutely normal. My pregnancy was a terrible ordeal, with bed rest for the last couple of months, round-the-clock monitoring, tubes of meds hooked to me, even a speed dial to the nursing staff, in case I had too many contractions within any hour. I was constantly on pins and needles. In fact, I am still waiting for some word from my higher power that I can relax and enjoy my miracle—and my son is five years old!"

Carolyn echoes the same reassurance.

"I thought that once I got past fourteen weeks I'd be able to relax—that was the point when my one and only other pregnancy ended—but I was wrong," she writes. "I still worried about everything, movement or no movement, symptoms or no symptoms. I finally decided that I was not going to allow infertility to rob me of the joy that should come with pregnancy. I forced myself to shut out bad thoughts and focus on the positive. It was a constant battle, but I was able to calm down after a while. I kept reminding myself that I really could not do any more than I was already doing to ensure a happy outcome. The result is now seven years old!"

This theme of mistrust is a common and recurring phenomenon throughout such hard won pregnancies. Many pregnant women who have battled with infertility will tell you that they feel their pregnancies are somehow predestined to fail. They have had so much failure in the past that they can't quite believe any other outcome is possible.

Other Emotional Repercussions

Sometimes the sense of impending tragedy or failure and the resulting emotional tumult during pregnancy may emanate from experiences other than infertility. For my patient, Candace, a decision that she'd made to terminate a pregnancy when she was very young continued to haunt her.

"I was fifteen and a sophomore in high school when I got pregnant and had an abortion," she told me. "I didn't ever want to walk that path again, so to protect myself from another unplanned pregnancy, I had an IUD put in. Years later, I learned that the string attached to the IUD created a silent infection in my womb that caused significant scarring. I needed surgery to clean up the area and remove the IUD. Two years later, I had to be operated on again for a ruptured ovarian cyst. Now, here I am at forty, finally in a solid relationship, ready and trying to become pregnant, and I can't. I've begun thinking again about the child I never had. Perhaps this is God's way of punishing me. I'm afraid I'll never be able to have a baby."

Although Candice did, in fact, eventually become pregnant, her generalized feelings of doom did not abate. I recommended that she see a therapist to gain insight into why her feelings were so persistent and continued to have such power over her life. In time, Candice discovered her negative emotions were due to unresolved feelings from the circumstances surrounding her abortion. She was able to gain a new perspective through her adult eyes and accept that as a teenager she'd had few options other than the one she had chosen as a single, pregnant girl without adequate family support who would have had to drop out of school to care for her baby and herself. She learned to grieve her earlier loss and move on with a more compassionate understanding of the issues she'd faced as a teenager.

Another type of emotional fallout that expectant ART parents may experience is a feeling of guilt about their growing need for privacy as they make their way through pregnancy and the eventual disclosure process. Katja clearly describes these "push, pull" misgivings in her message to the women in MVED-L.

"Yesterday, at Christmas, we told my husband's family that we were pregnant. (I am 19 weeks via donor embryo). We are not telling them the whole truth at this point, and I feel so guilty. They were all so happy! On the one hand, I don't think they would understand. On the other hand, I feel horrible keeping the secret from them.

"I did not have counseling beforehand. My clinic did not recommend any therapy, and I thought I could handle everything, no problem. I just jumped right in, not thinking about things like telling/not telling, genetic links, or anonymous donor issues. I don't mean to scare anyone out there who is currently trying to become pregnant, but I hope that you will think about all these issues before and maybe talk to someone about them. I am talking to a counselor now, but I still have a lot to sort out about everything."

Like Katja, I feel that I, too, would have benefited greatly from counseling when I began my journey into ART. When I first read her online message and advice, it resonated very strongly for me and became one of the primary reasons that I decided to write this book.

Prenatal Care and Confidentiality

It may be tempting, for a number of reasons, for expectant mothers to withhold their ART history from their doctors, but I strongly advise against it. Some women fear, in spite of assurances of patient confidentiality, that their doctors might inadvertently include an ART notation in a prenatal chart, later to be read by others, or make a verbal slip in front of the delivery or newborn nursery staff after the baby is born. Despite these concerns, I would urge all prenatal patients to share with their obstetricians—and later, with their pediatricians—their full health history, including what ART procedures were necessary for conception.

There are safeguards available. Mothers can ensure that disclosure be strictly limited to their obstetrician and pediatrician by asking that no recognizable ART notations be made in either the prenatal or pediatric records. A codified form of the ART data (similar to what we already have in place for HIV testing) can be entered onto the chart in a manner that insures that no one, other than the treating physicians, will be able to identify or access the contents of the confidential data.

Prior to delivery, a mother and her obstetrician should discuss the possibility of a different doctor attending the delivery if the primary doctor is unavailable when she goes into labor. If this happens, it might be useful for the primary doctor to make all pertinent notations on her chart in advance so that an on-call doctor reviewing the chart can be reassured that all appropriate prenatal screening was offered and discussed with the patient. One example of a pertinent notation for any prenatal patient over the age of 34 years would be that genetic amniocentesis was discussed and offered, but that the patient elected not to have it performed. The reason need not be described, but the covering physician will know that the test hadn't been overlooked and can proceed with that reassurance.

Some parents wonder why they should tell the pediatrician anything at all about their baby's conception. It is my firm belief that all IVF/ART children should be carefully followed by their pediatricians in a manner that protects the confidentiality wishes of the parents, but that can be tracked for purposes of quality of care. If medicine should discover at some future time that ART children are at any increased risk for certain health conditions or anomalies, pediatricians would want to be able to identify these children and communicate with their parents so that any ongoing health needs are appropriately screened for and addressed in a timely manner.

This lesson was learned in the case of diethylstilbestrol (DES), a drug used years ago to treat women at increased risk for miscarriage in early pregnancy when the fetus was still developing. It wasn't until the daughters of these DES mothers reached adulthood that long-term health risks were discovered that required careful monitoring, in some cases even intervention, to protect them from developing a rare form of cervical cancer. The good news is that this rare cancer could be screened for, once we knew where to look for the problem.

The Little Stranger Inside

There's no single road map for carrying an ART baby to whom you don't have a genetic link. Expectant mothers can worry: "Will my baby like me?" "Maybe I won't smell right." "What if I can't bond with my baby?"

For me, it hardly seemed logical that while carrying a child so intimately connected to me through my hopes and dreams, a child that was also a part of a man I'd loved for more than twenty-six years, I would imagine that I might not "know" this child at all. But there it was, the disconcerting thought that when this baby arrived, he might be totally an unknown to me. I never had such thoughts before my other children were born. Although I was certain my first child would be a girl and my second a boy, and in both instances I was wrong, that fact didn't trouble me in the least. So why would my "not knowing" this child be so disconcerting?

Inherent in my thinking was the assumption that if you "know" your child, you will have an instinctive and unbreakable bond to enjoy for all time. The unknown for me was the presence of the donor in my body and in my child, a presence that felt like an unpredictable virus. Would it somehow hurt us? I would never have thought twice about whether I could have bonded with an adopted child. So, what was different about this experience that I just couldn't get my mind entirely around it?

I believe, as I look back, it was the simple fact that there existed no historical precedent for what I was doing. I had no idea how to embrace my donor as a part of me and of my child. My journey was into the unknown, into a world where our science goes marching boldly forth, without adequate psychic preparation. I had no paradigm for it.

Other mothers by donor ovum and donor embryo have also had difficulty initially relating to the little strangers they carried inside, but they all found that the strangeness was soon eclipsed as a result of the love that invariably grows for their developing child.

"I know how it feels to wonder if you will bond with your baby," Joyce acknowledges in the chat room at MVED-L, "but now I say there is no question about it! You will be protective and all the other things a mother is to her child . . . for the rest of your life. True, your child will never have your eyes or your hair, but these genetic histories become less relevant over time. I've had to answer the question from moms in the playground, 'Where does he get those eyes?' And the truth is, they're from a person I don't know and my son will never know. It bothers me, but less and less as the years pass, and I'd do it all over again to have him."

Keahi, another mother by anonymous ovum donation, offers online reassurance to a pregnant woman who is struggling to find peace with the loss of the genetic link to her fetus. "If you have fears that maybe you won't love or accept this child, you can put those fears aside," she writes. "I, too, worried about how I would feel about a child that was not genetically mine, and for a long time I felt that genetics was very important. But from the first moment I found out I was pregnant, and even more so at my daughter's birth and with every day that goes by, I can't even describe to you how much I love her, how much she is ours, and I wonder why did I ever have those fears and wait so long. I don't think there are any parents of ovum donor children who would want any other kids but the ones who so miraculously have been given to them. I hope that by reading this, it convinces you that it is definitely the right thing, and you will never be sorry."

Cassie adds her wholehearted agreement. "I love my baby boy more than life itself. I promise you, the minute you get your baby in your arms, and they say 'Congratulations Mom!' all the fears and doubts about yourself and your baby not being genetically linked will just melt away. I think we tend to love these miracle babies so intensely because of all we've endured to get them! I also have genetic kids (grown), and this little guy we were given is just a total gift!"

Nanette's perspective takes a wider, historical view that has brought her total peace of mind. "I remember going into a church in Limerick, Ireland and seeing an inscription on a crypt: 'Fifteen years a maiden, one year a wife, two weeks a mother, then I left this life.' That was the reality for most women then, repeatedly risking death and/or watching your children die, and, even today, it is the reality for women in a large part of the world. And even in America, these tragedies can still happen.

"So when I look into my son's face, I don't scan his eyebrows or his chin or anything else to see if there might be the slightest resemblance to me as a little girl. I see that I am alive and healthy (and I would have been dead if medical science could not have delivered him safely by C-section) and I see that he is alive and healthy and not physically or mentally challenged, as so many children are. He is not going to die, as so many children used to, because he got an infected finger or a fever or appendicitis or one of a hundred other things that a doctor can now fix in a minute. And boy, that is good enough for me. I'm not asking God for one thing more."

Whether it's a mother who suddenly sees her husband's yawn in her newborn infant, or the mom and dad who travel miles to a foreign land to set eyes for the first time on their adopted toddler, or the anxious parent who searches for recognition in the eyes of her newborn, the bonding instinct is an ancient insurance package that mother nature programs into all living beings to help assure survival. A sense of family and belonging inevitably develops, regardless of genes.

The Magic Moment: Delivery

In all my years of practicing medicine, I've come to believe that the two most profound events that can be shared with another human being are birth and death. They are times like no others, and it is a great and precious privilege to be in attendance at these passages in and out of life.

In our modern, technologically sophisticated world, we have insulated ourselves from conscious acceptance of our inevitable departing so thoroughly that death is often approached with fear and distrust. But anyone who has had the opportunity to be with a loved one (or a patient) at the time of death may understand the privilege of which I speak. It is a heightened ephemeral moment in time that paradoxically lasts forever. When your dying loved one is made comfortable and kept as aware as possible, unusual opportunities may be created.

My brother and sister and I were all with my mother at the time of her death. She was quite short of breath near the end, and I was able to adjust her morphine drip until I saw the furrow between her brows start to soften. While her favorite music played quietly from a small cassette player by her head, I lay down beside her, spooning myself against her aged, frail back, and began to speak the most important words I would ever say to her.

First, I told her that she was not alone. We, her three children, were all there with her. Then I asked her to thank her body for the wonderful journey it had carried her on over the years. Next I asked her if I might create a picture for to hold in her mind. (She had been a talented painter.)

When she nodded, I asked her to visualize herself lying upon the soft white feathered back of a giant bird. With each breath she took in, the bird's wings would lift her up, and with each exhalation, the wings would descend. With every release of breath, all the tiredness she felt would go out from her. After a few seconds of this, I had the giant bird fly her to all the special places I knew she had visited and loved during her life: the place of her birth and childhood, the home of her marriage where she had lived and raised us, the countries to which she had traveled while my father was alive, and finally the home of her later years and the garden she'd loved so much. As the journey progressed, I watched her brow continue to relax. Soon after the story was over, she took in her last breath and let it go without the slightest protest.

You might ask, what has this to do with birth? The answer is: to me, everything.

Once labor starts, especially in the second stage when the baby begins to descend through the pelvis, a mother must push with all the force of a thousand generations before her, for she knows, at some primal level, that her child is dying until the outside—and freedom—can be reached. The baby must arrive in time to allow the return of circulation through the umbilical cord and to allow that first breath of much needed air that will restart the proper functioning of all the physiological systems.

Our transition into life outside the womb is as pivotal and intimate a moment as is our transition into death, each event marked by a single breath. Both death and birth happen naturally and don't necessarily require any intervention, and both can be lonely and frightening experiences. But neither experience needs to be either lonely or frightening. I believe it is our responsibility, whenever we attend a death or a birth, to provide reassurance, to encourage a willingness to go forward. I found the gentle journey of my mother's passing, with those who loved her in close attendance, to have much in common with the gentle journey of entry into the world as advocated by the French obstetrician, Frederic Leboyer.

Leboyer believes that an infant's entry into the world should be quiet and without struggle as much as possible. He advocates a gentle birth method, easing the transition from intra-uterine to extra-uterine life by leaving the umbilical cord intact so that the newborn has the benefit of oxygenated cord blood passing through his body, in addition to the first breaths of air filling the lungs. Once breathing is well established, the cord eventually stops pulsating and can be tied off. I started performing deliveries in this way in Boston in the 1970s and found them to be some of the most emotionally rewarding experiences I would ever have as a physician. I was soon to apply what I had learned to my personal life, as well.

My Story: Dauber, Jessica, and Tucker

Our first child, Dauber, was four when we decided to try and have another. During my second pregnancy, there were times when I became extremely wistful, thinking that soon a unique chapter in our family lives would be closing. Our first born would no longer be our only child, and I started to imagine what it would be like to share time that had been exclusively his and mine with a younger sibling. I found myself in a kind of subtle mourning. I was even reluctant to pick out a name for the new baby, as if that brought the reality of a sibling closer to home. I would play with and pat the little munchkin inside, but name her, I just couldn't.

It was critically important to me during the pregnancy that our son, Dauber, be excited and happy about having a little sister or brother. I started to prepare him so that the transition would be as easy as possible. So, it came as no surprise when he blithely announced one day to his nursery school teacher that he would be helping his mommy and daddy "borne my little sister." From then on it was impossible for me to even consider excluding him from the delivery. Please understand that this was back in the 1970's, when it was still considered radical to have a family birth with siblings present. The psychiatric community was conflicted about whether or not a young child witnessing birth might suffer emotional harm because he would see his mother in "such pain."

To address these concerns, we brought our son to all our La Maze classes and were careful to make loud and dramatic grunting noises during pushing practice to prepare him for the real thing. We also showed him the movies we had taken of his own birth so he would know what to expect. After all, birth is a messy business, and we didn't want him to think blood and other body fluids were signs of anything going wrong. We also had to release the hospital of any liability, as well as obtain a pediatrician's clearance.

Our daughter's entrance into the world followed a short labor. Her birth was fast and slippery, and our son's reaction, to our delight, was quite matter of fact. As a result, perhaps, of his experience at the delivery, he soon developed a possessive attitude towards his baby sister, regarding her as something new and exciting in his world, rather than someone with whom he would have to compete for my attention.

I'd say our son's preparation was an unmitigated success. I also believe that the efforts I made on his behalf were really more about me than him. I found that by preparing my son, I could bond with my daughter following birth without feeling that loving either of my children was like dipping water from a finite well.

As soon as my daughter was safely out of me, we didn't over-stimulate her to get her to cry, but instead placed her on my abdomen and covered her with a pre-warmed towel. I gently massaged her torso and watched carefully as she started spontaneously to breathe. Her cord was still open between us and pulsating, sending her oxygenated blood, as I breathed deeply in and out, sending her more oxygen from my own circulation—all standard procedure with the Leboyer method.

Tucker's delivery was a bit different. First of all, his brother, Dauber, was then twenty-three years old. He helped me with my pushing, coaching me through the bars of the delivery bed. My husband, David, was giving me expert counter pressure on my lower back, where I was feeling plenty of pain. My daughter, Jessica, then eighteen, was keeping a careful eye out for the anesthesiologist who seemed to be taking his own sweet time arriving to give me an epidural. Tucker was stuck in my mid pelvis, and I thought an epidural would allow his head to descend through the cervix in better alignment.

Finally, in exasperation with all the waiting and pain, I yelled though the delivery room door, "Get that #%*#@*% anesthesiologist in here right now!" Amazingly, he appeared immediately and gave me the relief I had been waiting for.

The epidural worked like a charm; Tucker's head descended right to the perineum. I listened to the monitor and heard his heart beat slowing and not recovering. And then I started to push, with everyone around me sensing the urgency and calling out to me to push harder, harder. And then, out he came, all limp. My obstetrician offered to place him on my belly as we had planned, but I said, "No way, you get him started, right now. He needs support."

It seemed like forever until I heard that first cry, and I believe none of us took a breath until Tucker did. My daughter, Jessica, took him over to the warm bassinette, and under the watchful eye of the nurse, wiped him down and put on his little knit cap. She brought him to me as soon as he was stable. That was when we turned down the lights and placed him in a basin of warm water that had been previously prepared. I supported his head, allowing the rest of his body to float free. He immediately settled into the water, his limbs curling into their womb positions, his face full of pure curiosity as he peered with wide eyes into the darkened room where he heard our hushed and happy voices.

Like Dauber's presence at his sister's birth, the presence of both Dauber and Jessica at Tucker's birth was something I encouraged more for me than for them. This time, I needed the reassurance that they would fully accept their new sibling, that they would not feel resentment toward him, nor toward me for wanting to have another child and for going to such lengths to have him.

Tucker's birth was as beautiful and ended as peacefully as I could ever have wanted or imagined. Like all births, it was unique and special, and yet it was also just another note in the endless, magic symphony of the human experience.

A Lesson in Etiquette

During Tucker's delivery, every member of my "team" contributed in his or her own way to ensure the physical safety and emotional well being of mother and child—just as it should be in all deliveries. Unfortunately, things do not always go that way.

Recently, an ART parent shared with me her pain at the memory of a thoughtless and inappropriate comment that was made immediately after the birth of her baby and that burned her to the core. She was in the delivery room, in stirrups, with a sore bottom from her stitches, when she overheard her sister say to her mother who was also present, "Oh, doesn't the baby have Nina's eyes!" Nina was the ovum donor, a close relative known to both sister and mother of the patient. Where these family members get their social IQ's I can't imagine. This is a good example of the kind of discussion that should never occur around new parents.

It is a privilege for anyone to be invited to attend the miracle of birth or to visit new parents and their newborn in the hospital. But all visitors should know—or have it spelled out for them in advance, if need be—that every parent has the right to experience the joy of giving birth without any reminders about the help or contributions of sperm or ovum donors interfering with their special first moments of bonding with their baby.

It is the responsibility of everyone in attendance at a birth to know the boundaries that come with his or her role in the delivery and to behave accordingly, especially where the pregnancy involves ART. This includes physicians and other health care personnel. They as much as anyone need to be sensitive to the vulnerability of ART parents, to understand and appreciate the incredible journey ART parents undertook to reach the intimate moment of birth, and to avoid thoughtless or hurtful comments or questions.

Chapter 7

Bringing Baby Home

Given all that you've been through, when you finally arrive home with baby in arms, is it any wonder you can't quite believe it's true? Suddenly, everything has changed, and your life will never be the same. For all new parents, even those who had no difficulty in achieving a successful pregnancy, there is an inevitable period of adjustment with the newest and tiniest family member taking over the household.

All babies are different and respond differently to their parents. These differences may be due to any number of things that have nothing whatsoever to do with genetics. Some babies are lively and active, apparently fascinated by faces from their first moments, with eyes that follow movement constantly whenever they are awake. Others appear more sleepy and less interested in what is going on around them. But no matter what sort of demeanor or "personality" your baby appears to have during the early weeks of life, the bonding that perhaps you feared might not occur *will* occur and will steadily grow, prompted not just by nature, which programs this bonding process into all mothers to insure survival of the species, but especially reinforced for ART moms as a result of the extraordinary love and sacrifices that brought their babies to them.

Our first baby, a big-eyed boy, was calm and quiet, studying everything in the room with what appeared to be mild curiosity. But his eyes were always looking off in the distance rather than focusing on me. I felt a responsive, urgent, need to place myself directly into his line of vision, trying to establish a pathway for human recognition.

Our second baby was quite different, constantly in motion. Interested mostly in the tactile experience of nursing, she would first stare right at the breast in front of her, almost cross-eyed, and then try to get a good grip on my skin with her tiny hand. Her eyes seemed to seek me out, back and forth between breast and face, while she suckled, all the while patting or batting at the breast with her little fists.

Our third little one, Tucker, preferred to nestle quietly in my arms while he was feeding, as long as he could reach up with his tiny fingers to stroke my eyelashes. He did this every time he nursed, and it fascinated me and gave me great joy and peace. I found it amazing that he never once stuck his finger in my eye.

In the past, some family counselors who received their training prior to the availability of ART, wondered, as did their infertile clients, whether there might be a less intense bond experienced by an ART parent whose child does not share his or her genetics. And they considered how best to address issues that might interfere with parental bonding, especially in ART families with children of mixed origins. Time has proven, however, that those concerns were unfounded; they simply have *not* been borne out by the general ART experience.

As with all new relationships, parent/child bonding for some new mothers occurs immediately, while such bonding for other mothers takes more time. This is absolutely normal. What is important to remember is that bonding with our babies can be an immediate sensation of oneness or it can be a gently unfolding process, starting out tentatively and building in its intimacy over weeks. The chemistry of the process does not depend on genetic sameness between parent and infant to be successful.

The Ties that Bind

In the chat room at MVED-L, the shared experiences about bonding are abundant. New mothers love to tell their happy tales of bringing their babies home and discovering the intense joys of parenthood. It is one of the most popular topics for discussion, and it inspires hope in everyone to hear such rich and wonderful success stories. Here's a sampling:

Marsha: Learning about Patience and Trust

"Everything happened so fast with my delivery, I had no time to react. I was standing at the kitchen sink when I felt a warm gush. Dennis was just coming in the driveway and found me on the phone frantically trying to reach our doctor. 'My waters broke! And there's something down there.' I was terrified the baby was already coming. But that was not what happened. Instead, as we learned in the ambulance, our daughter's cord had prolapsed. We were in a real emergency. All I remember from then on was being whisked into the operating room to have a Caesarean. That's how Sarah came into our lives, weighing one and a half pounds.

"She looked so fragile all hooked up to tubes in the ICU. A ventilator was assisting her breathing and a feeding tube was placed in her stomach since she was too weak to suck on her own. All I could do was stroke her tummy and let her feel the tip of my finger in her tiny grasp. Looking at her, all ruddy and velvet skinned, I kept thinking she would never survive. Dennis was able to stay with her, thank God. I couldn't stand to stay long. In a state of numbness, I went from day to day, recovering from my surgery until it was time for me to go home. Sarah stayed on, of course. I found, as the days turned to weeks, that I could only visit her briefly. I felt so guilty; my body and spirit had just given out, and I found myself sleeping more and more, spacing out my visits to the hospital. But Sarah hung in there, fighting for her life.

"I felt like such a failure as a mother. Why couldn't I stay with her? Dennis stood by both of us. Whenever he wasn't with Sarah, he was with me, telling me to take the time I needed to heal, just as Sarah was doing.

"Well, we eventually made it. Sarah is home now, and at five and a half pounds, she's our little angel. She has taught me so much about patience and trust. It took me so long to believe she would live, and I understand now how terrified I was to feel close to her. But, you know, you have no choice, the closeness just happens in spite of your worries."

Ginny: Instant Bonding

"I remember when my first child was born, a son. I'd shielded myself from my feelings somewhat. He was my third try at DE, and I didn't feel the ice start to break right away. My pregnancy was great, but the delivery was quite difficult. I had a C-section, following many hours of exhausting labor.

"After I was back in the room, they brought him to me, and I looked at him dispassionately. 'Who are you?' I wondered. 'Do you look like her?' I wasn't sure how I felt about that little stranger. I was looking at him, trying to sort out my feelings and hoping I could come to love him. Then he yawned. It was my husband's yawn, and I fell totally, instantly in love and haven't looked back."

Pamela: Mom by Adoption and by Ovum Donation

"I didn't originally have a name for the kind of parenting I have taken on, but I guess I might call it 'attachment style parenting,' a new term for me. I am learning about this as I go.

"The whole issue started over the adoption of my daughter. As healthy as she is, I know that she is wired differently from many children who have had the opportunity to immediately bond with their birth or adoptive parents. She is bright, outgoing, and happy and appears very smart, but under it all, she is very sensitive to my husband's and my moods. After the birth of her brother by ovum donation last month, I realized how sensitive she is and recognized her need for more physical contact with my husband and me.

"She needed to return to our room to sleep with us (our room, her bed). So now the four of us are in one room. Since then, I have worked to attune myself more to her needs. I know she needs consistency, calmness, humor, and lots of physical contact. In international adoptions, some children come from orphanages, but others, like our daughter, come from foster families. So my daughter had bonded with her foster mom, and now had to re-bond with us. There are techniques for assisting the bonding process, but unfortunately the agency did not pass these on to us.

"I and other adoptive moms have had to discover and create as we go along. It's almost like recreating an infant's bonding experience! I initially felt a tremendous urge to breast-feed my daughter. I did try, initially, but could not get my new eight-month old to become interested. Luckily, this time around, I have been able to nurse our son from birth. And our daughter is getting an infusion of snuggle time, much to everyone's delight."

Very often we see older siblings responding similarly to Pamela's older adopted daughter at the time of a new sibling's birth. An older child may seek reassurance and express a need for increased contact, especially at night. This is often manifested by a desire to share the parental room, especially if an infant's crib is located there. Pamela has shown an endearing sensitivity to the needs of her older child at a time of intimate adjustment for the whole family.

Holly: Tying the Apron Strings

"Meg certainly tolerates our schedules better than we do. I'm in the third year of my pediatric residency, and my husband, Mason, has been preparing for his bar exam. When I'm on-call, Mason brings Meg in to the hospital so we can all spend the night together. As long as I'm not off in the emergency room, I can nurse her in the lounge and he can get time to study. It's a crazy life, I know, but we'd have it no other way. Meg is such a blessing.

"When Mason married me, he knew that I would be unable to have genetic children of my own. We were so lucky to have an ovum donor help us realize our dreams of having a family. Even now, I have the hardest time taking an instant of leisure time away from Meg! She's ten months old, yet I still can't get enough of her.

"I remember when she was just twelve weeks old, and Mason arranged for a neighbor to look after Meg so we could have our first evening out together. Everything was going just great, until I heard the sitter settling Meg into her crib. As I was listening to all those cooing noises, I found myself running into our bedroom where Mason was getting dressed. I threw myself onto our bed and burst into tears. 'I haven't even tied the apron strings yet, and now I have to share her!' I cried. I really hadn't expected such a strong reaction. But there you have it, one of the many aspects of being a new parent. We did eventually go out together that evening, and Meg's social life got off to a wonderful start with the sitter."

My Story: Sharing Tucker with Jessica

The bonding experience with Tucker for my family and me was atypical. Soon after he arrived home, his skin began to turn yellow, indicating a case of newborn jaundice.[35] This meant I had to take him back and forth to the hospital every day for painful heel sticks that nearly broke my heart. The best and worst of it, though, were yet to come.

We were instructed that because of his dangerously high bilirubin levels[36] he needed to sleep at night on a special mat of blue light that absorbed the damaging pigment accumulating in his skin. During his waking hours, he also had to remain under the "bili" lights, wearing protective shields over his eyes and genitals at all times. My daughter went a bit berserk over this, feeling the treatment, though necessary, was extremely cruel for her little brother to face in his early weeks of

---

[35] Newborn jaundice is a transient condition that can happen when a baby has an ABO blood incompatibility that produces too many products in his circulation for his liver to break down and process. If the products rise too high in the bloodstream, an exchange transfusion may be necessary to prevent brain damage.

[36] Bilirubin is one of the blood breakdown products that must be lowered to prevent brain damage.

life. It essentially closed him off in darkness, away from our smiling faces and the wonder of his new world.

The good part was that the nurses at the hospital, as a special favor to me, managed to help us locate and take home a set of bili lights to be set up in our bedroom. This was a highly unusual arrangement, a rare exception to the rule, and no small task, since we're talking here about a heavy, cumbersome unit, five feet high, with a hood of bright lights designed to shine down over a crib.

With the arrival of the equipment, our daughter went into high gear, pinning together a tent of sheets around the unit to capture the light, then arranging a kind of camp-bed set up underneath. She slept beside her baby brother during the day, whenever he napped, making sure his eye patches stayed on and that the protection between his legs remained in place. When he was awake, we would peek in to find her holding his tiny hand and quietly singing to him, massaging him or telling him stories. I had to get in line to get into that tent for my own exclusive time. Our little boy received constant touching and caressing during those early days, so that by the time he was ready to have his eye patches off for any significant period of time, the transition to his greater world would be smooth as silk. It was a bit of an ordeal, but it created special memories and forged new bonds for all of us.

The Solomon Syndrome

Occasionally, a woman who has struggled with infertility and becomes pregnant via ART will experience a frame of mind that is characterized by a sense of unworthiness. If it is not addressed, it can threaten the bonding process between mother and baby, and it can put her at risk for full-blown post partum depression. I call this frame of mind the "Solomon Syndrome."

In the Bible, when Solomon sought to resolve the issue of which of two women claiming to be an infant's mother was the genuine one, the real mother, upon learning that Solomon would cut the child in half, said that the child belonged to the other woman. The moral of the story, of course, is that a real mother will do whatever is necessary to secure the safety and well being of her offspring. What more dramatic proof is there than to give up what is yours, if that is what must be, in order that your child may survive or find happiness?

A mother via ovum donation who feels that she nurtures a little stranger within her body may struggle with feelings of inadequacy and unworthiness. Shaken in her self-confidence by her journey through infertility, this mother might worry that her baby will not find her good enough. An intense sadness may well up in her as she imagines her child wishing for its "genetic mother," its "real mother." She may wonder if it would be better to give up her child to her donor, imagining that the child will prefer the love and acceptance of this "other mother."

Such a frightening fantasy can consume whatever vestiges of self-confidence the pregnant mother has, so that by the time of the birth, she feels she must somehow make this "donor mother" available to her baby, to be loved by her child, whatever the cost of the loss to her. As she anticipates what she feels will be an inevitable future loss, she becomes increasingly saddened and hesitant to initiate bonding behavior. Her devastating fantasy places her in an emotionally vulnerable position, particularly during the first four to six weeks of the newborn's life, when parents' nurture of their baby has yet to be rewarded by a smile of recognition! Add a good case of colic to the mix, and she may have even more convincing evidence that her inconsolable newborn does not find her adequate to meet his needs.

For a woman suffering from this syndrome, there is much that can be done. A father's involvement, for example, can make a big difference to the success of the bonding process between mother and infant.

"We have taken this path together for no other reason than to bring this wonderful baby into our family," he might gently remind his wife. "No one knows better than we do how hard the journey has been. The one and only mother of our child is you, the one who has been willing and able to nurture this unique young life from a bundle of cells into a fully formed human being. Without your desire and the fortitude to carry it through, our child would never otherwise be. Our donor is a partial genetic contributor, a kind woman, a giving woman, yes, but a mother to our child, no. She did not give either of us a child. Her contribution, a life giving cell, would have been passed out of her body, as have all her other life giving cells each month, but this time the cell was harvested and saved rather than passed on, and only because we needed it."

Such words can go a long way in erasing the maternal fantasy that somehow a baby will not find his mother good enough.[37] However, if fears of rejection and inadequacy persist, then professional counseling should be sought as soon as possible to stop the cascade of ideas that places the mother at risk for a full-blown post partum depression.

Post Partum Depression

Post partum depression can strike without warning, even weeks or months after delivery, and the signs, symptoms, and risk factors are often minimized or overlooked. With the sudden drop in hormones following delivery, the sleepless nights, and the stress of caring for a newborn, all mothers are at risk to some degree. Women who have had prior episodes of depression or a family history of depressive disorders are at increased susceptibility. Because of the unique stresses associated with long-standing infertility, and then the ongoing difficult decisions parents must make as they pursue ART, it comes as no surprise that the risk is heightened for this group of women, as well.

Post partum depression can occur as late as six to twelve months following even the most uneventful delivery. All prenatal patients, their partners, and their advocates should know what to look for. The

---

[37] Single mothers without a partner for support are just as susceptible to the same destructive fantasies of the Solomon Syndrome. It is important that single mothers have a support person available throughout pregnancy, delivery, and the postpartum period. She might choose either a knowledgeable family member, or someone who has also been through assisted conception.

blues are commonly experienced as episodic weepiness and fatigue. But it's not a case of "just the blues" if a mother experiences:

- insomnia
- a sense of hopelessness or panic about the wellbeing of herself or her family,
- difficulty performing simple tasks
- withdrawal from normal family activities she used to enjoy.

Depression is a serious matter. It is real and it is debilitating. Professional help is needed if any of these symptoms occur and persist for more than a week. If, in the first weeks and months following birth, you should find yourself becoming agitated, unable to sleep, losing the ability to care for your baby, slipping into a state of mind where life doesn't seem worth living, or harboring suicidal thoughts, you must get help immediately. Scientology is *not* the answer! Antidepressant/anti-anxiety medication is particularly effective, along with therapy. Don't try to handle it on your own. There is a way to work through it, even though you may be convinced that the situation is hopeless. In fact, a sense of hopelessness and guilt are classic hallmarks of postpartum depression.

My Story: Depression and Recovery

At five weeks postpartum, life seemed to be going along quite well. Tucker had recovered from his jaundice without requiring any transfusions, and we were starting to enjoy his new ability to truly smile. Our older children were getting ready to return to school back east. We had planned a farewell dinner for each of them at their restaurants of choice. Our son's farewell dinner came first, and I recall that I had macadamia nut crusted mahi mahi, followed by crème brulee. The next night, we set out to eat at a Mexican restaurant with our daughter and one of her best friends, who planned to drive her to the airport afterwards.

While we were waiting to be served our meals, I experienced a sudden and overwhelming sense of doom. I excused myself from the table and made a beeline for the restrooms. Splashing cold water on my face had no effect. There was a pay phone nearby. I pulled out some change and made an emergency call to a friend, a psychiatrist, to tell her what was happening.

Just then, my daughter came by and saw that there were tears running down my face. She stopped for a moment and told me not to feel bad or worry about her leaving. "Just look up at the ceiling, Mom," she said. "It's hard to cry when you're looking up, you know."

The remainder of the dinner was a blur. I struggled to maintain my composure, but by the time we hugged the girls goodbye, I was coming apart. "We have got to get me some help, right now!" I told David the moment we were alone. "Something is terribly wrong."

We immediately drove to my friend's home. It was hard for me to articulate anything of what I was experiencing; I had become essentially mute. She encouraged me to get more rest and to check in with her if things didn't improve after a good night's sleep. Over the next few days, I slipped in and out of an extreme anxiety state without warning. It was time to get a complete medical evaluation. I knew something was going very wrong, but I had no idea what it was.

At first my doctors seemed stumped. My blood pressure began to skyrocket in intervals up to dangerous levels, my face would become flushed and my pupils enlarged. I was tested for everything from thyroid storm to adrenal tumors. No one believed me when I said I thought I was going insane. Perhaps they thought that anyone who was able to provide her own diagnosis couldn't be really and truly crazy.

Fortunately, my psychiatrist friend listened to what I was saying and took me seriously. She started me on anti-depressants, and I saw her regularly for about 18 months. My husband, David, was a tremendous support, as were family members and friends. Mine was a classic, severe case of post-partum depression. Although it was quite debilitating for the first several months, I did not need to be hospitalized and was able to function normally most of the time, despite episodes of intense despair. After about six months, my symptoms were less severe and sporadic, and after a year and a half, I was back to my old self.

The Reality of Parenthood

Here's a secret every parent knows: In loving the child you have, no matter how parenthood was achieved, you will find that it is hard to imagine loving the next child as much. But this idea is really no more than smoke, as the following stories reveal.

Hillary: "Don't Over Analyze"

"We had three children, two sons and a daughter, during the first ten years of our marriage, and then our family building was on hiatus while my husband went through a major career change. Our children were such good kids, always quiet and well behaved. They never gave us any problems beyond the occasional twisted ankle or run to the emergency room for stitches. We really lucked out.

"When we decided to try to have another child, I was in my 40's, and I kept miscarrying due to old eggs. This was a shock. I'd been so fertile, I never thought I'd have trouble getting pregnant, but I miscarried five times.

"Going to donor ovum was also something I thought I would never do. All I could think of was how perfect our older kids had turned out, how could we ever hope to be as lucky with a donor? We very carefully chose the donor, and she was an excellent match. We were on her waiting list and about to be the next recipients when the clinic called to say she had hyper-stimulated on her previous cycle, produced only one egg, and was dropping out of the program. Because we were ready to go, the clinic offered us another donor. She was a wonderful choice, but with very different qualities than our first choice. After adjusting our sights, we said okay.

"I got pregnant on our first try and had a little boy! He couldn't be more perfect or more loved. It's difficult to even speak of how much we love him without getting emotional, we are absolutely nuts about this child. I'm sure others get tired of hearing us carrying on!

"So here we are trying again for a little sibling. We have nine remaining embryos from the previous IVF procedure, but I am beside myself thinking about what will we do if we need to make multiple tries at pregnancy and use up all the embryos. Our donor is now out of the program, and I'm panicked at the thought of having to use another donor. How could we possibly come up with a donor who will help us produce another child as perfect and delightful as our son?

"Of course, I see the irony. Here I am asking the same questions that I had in the beginning when considering a donor ovum: How can a child conceived with a donor possibly compare to our biological kids? And, then again, how could another child possibly compare to the perfect child from our previous donor?

"I know everyone must work these things out for themselves, but sometimes I wonder if the best advice is simply: Don't think so much, don't over-analyze, just have a baby and love him. It's impossible not to."

Remi: Thoughts on Genetics

"The emptiness and pain of childlessness has given way to the chaos, joy, frustration, and the utter fullness of life as a mother of thirteen-month-old boy/girl twins, whom I love more than anything in the world. These two little souls are an incredible gift. I could not care less whose genetics they carry. They are my children!

"I watch them grow and develop, laugh and cry, sleep and wake, and I cannot believe that I ever considered the loss of my genetics an issue. Instead, I am overjoyed that these are my children.

"I don't spend time any more looking for myself in them. I like to think that I appreciate my kids for who they are and will become and will not try to pigeonhole them into any preconceived notions of whom they ought to be, based on their heritage. I used an anonymous donor, so their talents, looks, skills, personalities and interests will be new to me, and I'm thrilled about it! It's one long discovery process for all of us. And we enjoy watching it unfold every single day.

"These days, since I've experienced motherhood, the idea of requiring a genetic link to have a loving relationship with your children seems like the height of vanity to me! I take no credit for my kids' genetics, but you can bet I am as proud of them as I can possibly be!"

Melanie: The Irony of Looks

"Yes, I used to get a tug because our son is such a clone of his dad. But, after talking to other moms whose kids were clones of their dads and whom, I'm assuming, were not DE babies, I came to the realization that if I'd given him my chromosomes, he'd still look just like his daddy. I'd still have total strangers take one look at him and at me and say that he really looks a lot like his dad.

"Ironically, I think the sting is easing because this time around our daughter, also by DE, just happens to look so much like me. Strangers look at her and say she's mine. But I no longer scan my children's faces for traces of anyone. Instead, I'm enjoying watching their unique personalities develop."

Rhonda: Seeing her Donor in her Son

"I wouldn't trade my baby for any other in the world. I wouldn't even change the fact that I did not have genetic children if I could, for it would mean that Mickey would not exist. To think that if every horrible minute of infertility had been different and I had conceived a genetic child, Mickey would not be—well, that is just totally unacceptable!!

"Yet I do still have other feelings sometimes. Since I know my donor, sometimes I wish I didn't, though I would not change one thing about my child—he's perfect as he is. But I know every look, quirk and talent that comes from my donor, and everyone else in the family does too! We often laugh about how many things Mickey does that are just plain his Aunty to a tee. Still, I know that I am the right mom for Mickey, that he is just where he was meant to be and so am I."

Megan: Finding Completion

"I look at my seven-year-old daughter via donor egg, and it never crosses my mind that she doesn't look like me—she just looks like exactly who she is. I never imagine a different child, she is my one and only, the product of my dreams, and I wouldn't change a thing about her. I don't miss my genetics, truly I don't. I never feel anything when I look at her but utter joy and immense gratitude. I really cannot believe that people might feel sad after actually giving birth and having their DE children. It's so much more than I ever expected. I was infertile and miserable, longing for a baby to hold for fifteen long years. Now I am a mother, my daughter is my joy; she's beautiful, kind and sweet. I can't imagine looking at her any differently than I do now, even if she were my clone!"

Bette: It's the Commitment that Counts

In an effort to sum it all up, a woman named Bette, writing in the chat room of MVED-L, pulls no punches and speaks the lesson so many step-parents and ART parents have learned so well.

"Adoption, donor sperm, donor egg, donor embryo, and step-parenting, too, all involve making a commitment to parent a human being who is not genetically related. These are all issues of 'someone else's child.' But the genetics have nothing to do with loving, bonding, nurturing, and raising a child; it's the commitment that counts.

"Most people know of at least one genetic parent who chose not to participate in parenting a child. Sometimes this happens through divorce or even death. Now, please pay attention, because this next bit is very important: The genetic relationship doesn't always hold people together.

"I know that's a shock for those who are still reeling from the blow of losing their ability to have their own genetic progeny; unfortunately it's the truth. There are people out there who simply aren't interested in or capable of making a lifelong commitment to a child, regardless of whether or not they are genetically related. That level of commitment is a choice each of us makes.

"The bottom line is: family is attitude. When you make a conscious decision to commit to a child, today, tomorrow, and forever, that's family. When you decide to love for the rest of your life, no matter what may happen, that's family.

"Families are built in lots of ways. Some people feel closer to friends than they do to blood relatives, and these adopted relationships become family. Our bonds to others can be steadfast—with or without genetic links. We are capable of stretching the boundaries of whom, why and how we will love. When we stretch our hearts to include the joy of loving 'someone else's child,' we are the ones who benefit.

"Does this mean that life is going to be easy? No, of course not! No matter how perfect the child—or the parent—there will always be those moments when the thought will arise: 'What was I thinking?' (This is likely to occur at least once or twice during labor, for example, and innumerable times during a child's adolescence.) But you get past those times and on to the next, and that's okay!

"So, let me repeat: Adoption, donor sperm, donor egg, donor embryo, and step-parenting all involve making a commitment to love another human being with no genetic relationship, but it's an attitude that creates family. We are all blessed with the privilege of sharing our lives with one another. It's okay to be scared. It's even better to be doing it."

Marlene: A Special Farewell

"I just wanted to say goodbye to this wonderful group of women at Mothers Via Egg Donation. I received so much support from so many of you over the past years. Thank you. Our one and only try with an egg donor failed last year and now that I look back, it was the best thing that ever happened to me. We adopted a beautiful, healthy, perfect baby boy four months ago, and he is the baby that was meant to be ours, there is no doubt about that. Adoption was our answer and I'll never ever regret it. Good luck to you all on your journey to become moms."

Chapter 8

Telling Children Their Stories

Although some might question whether or not ART children should know their roots, I personally have no doubt about it. I believe all children deserve to know about their genetic tapestry as part of the story of their birth. I believe they are entitled to clear and direct answers to two fundamentally important questions:

- Who is my mommy/daddy?
- What are my origins?

The Ethics Committee of the American Society for Reproductive Medicine (ASRM) states that it "is the recipient parents' choice whether to disclose the fact of donor gamete conception to their offspring," and I agree. I also concur wholeheartedly with the committee's reasoning in support of full disclosure: "Because of persons' fundamental interest in knowing their genetic heritage and the importance of their ability to make informed health care decisions in the future, [we] support disclosure about the fact of donation to children. [We] also support the gathering and storing of medical and genetic information that can be provided to offspring if they ask."[38]

---

[38] Ethics Committee of the American Society of Reproductive Medicine, "Informing Offspring of their Conception by Gamete Donation," *Fertility and Sterility*, Vol. 81, No. 3, March 2004.

The 2005 President of ASRM, Dr. Robert Schenken, Professor and Chair of the Department of Obstetrics and Gynecology at the University of Texas Health Science Center at San Antonio, has expressed the view that medical professionals "do not need to advocate disclosure or non-disclosure of children's donor egg conception. These kids' parents want to make the right decision for their families, and it is up to them to determine what to tell their children and when. We can help them by offering counseling and by developing information materials appropriate for children of different ages."[39] But, unfortunately, we have a long way to go before ART parents can do this easily and sensibly. The language we use in talking with children about human reproduction in general, and ART in particular, is so important that I've devoted this chapter to a thorough exploration of how parents can communicate with their children and respond to their questions at various developmental stages.

Finding the Way

The decisions about what to tell children about their genetic heritage, the circumstances of their conception, and the details of their delivery are personal decisions that belong to parents and that all parents must make, not just ART parents. Some parents with a notorious ancestor who is an embarrassment to them might choose to omit mentioning this ancestor when discussing the family tree. Some parents are comfortable telling their children about "the night we made you." (Our oldest son was conceived in the aft cabin of a sloop on a rough passage from Antigua to Barbuda, and we laugh about that as a family because of my propensity for sea sickness.) Some parents are far more private about these things. And some parents film the births of their children to share the event with them when they are older, while others feel this is inappropriate.

---

[39] Greenfield and Klock, "Disclosure Decisions Among Known and Anonymous Oocyte Donation Recipients," *Fertility and Sterility*, Vol. 81, No. 6, June 2004.

For ART parents, the disclosure issues, particularly regarding genetic origins and conception, are more complex. Before deciding what to disclose, and when and how to make the disclosure, ART parents should ask themselves the following questions:

- If I were in my child's shoes, what would I want to know about myself, and when would I want to know it?
- In making our decision to disclose or not to disclose, are we distinguishing between our needs and those of our child?
- Are my husband and I of like mind on the disclosure issue? If not, how do we plan to resolve our differences?
- Are we ready to disclose material to our child and/or, eventually, to others in a comfortable, matter-of-fact way?
- Have we thought out what levels of detail are necessary to disclose to our child, and if so, at what ages will we say what?
- Are we comfortable with our child communicating what he/she learns to others?
- Can we visualize our child as an adult and a parent one day, feeling on solid ground about his/her origins?
- Do we have an integrated disclosure process for the other siblings too?

The Rewards of Openness

Carole Lieber Wilkins, a marriage and family therapist in Los Angeles, California has taught hundreds of people how to address these issues within their families. "Much of the time I find that fear of 'doing it wrong' or saying the wrong thing has paralyzed some parents into not saying anything," she reports. "But so far, no one who has been open with their children, families, and friends has come back to tell me they regretted it."

Lieber Wilkins is a mother through the use of ART herself and, with the wisdom that comes from experience, she goes on say: "While genetic relatedness is very important in the formation of a family, it is a paradox that it is also not at all important. Many people 'forget' my children are not genetically related to me and sometimes engage in that humorous conversation of trying to decide from whom the child may have inherited a particular quality from within my extended family before they remember or are reminded. This is done openly. My experience with non-family members who may have the information about donor egg is that they are initially intrigued because they have heard of it in the media, but probably don't know anyone who has done it. It is merely interesting, but I have *never* in 12 years received a comment that was hurtful. Once my children were here, they were real people, not identified by the circumstances of their births. Sometimes I have casually corrected a quirk of language by those not well-versed in unique family building, by adding the usual 'I am the real mother, that was our donor,' or other such positive language. Perhaps it is this casualness that sets the tone for acceptance from others, family or not. Yes, the cousins in our family are all cousins. They are black, white, and Asian, adopted, not adopted, easily conceived and mixed genetics. We are fortunate in that respect. But it goes without question. We are aware that we are unique, but family just the same."

For anyone who openly shares their methods of family building, as Lieber Wilkins has with her sons, the issue of the children hearing or learning about donor egg from someone else is moot. "Since they have grown up from the time of birth, from pre-verbal to verbal, hearing the language of our family building used often and casually in their home, there has never been a time when they did not hear, if not understand the 'different-ness' of our family," she says. "As time has gone on, they have understood in their own ways, at each developmental phase, what that different-ness means and what it means to them. As my infertility has taken a backseat in my own life, it comes more to the front seat for them. As they evaluate who they are in many ways, what was once very painful for me, the loss of my genetic offspring, has perhaps become meaningful to them. I consider it my job to make room for their feelings as they emerge."

Over the years, because of her work, Lieber Wilkins has talked with her sons about various disclosure issues, and the response is especially illuminating and reassuring for anyone who has worried about the consequences of openness.

"When I asked my younger son if his friends had ever talked with him about being conceived with a donor egg, his answer was, 'No! They wouldn't even know what to say cuz they don't understand it.' And how true," Lieber Wilkins remarks with bemusement. "What would an eight-year-old know about using another woman's ovum to obtain a pregnancy if his parents had not explained it as it relates to their own birth? Moreover, he has said to me: 'Nobody would care!' That has been my experience, too; no one cares. In addition to all of this, no one has the influence on children that parents do—no one. We set the tone. That may change as children develop their own thoughts or feelings about their genetic roots and may not like *not* being related genetically to their mom. That is the reality of the choice we made when we decided to bring them into our lives. That is the reality of their lives, and they will feel differently about it at different times."

Lieber Wilkins acknowledges that, like all parents, she has no doubt made mistakes with her children. "But the one thing I feel most proud of is setting a tone with my kids that they can always depend on me for the truth and there is nothing they cannot tell me," she says. "That is paying off a little as they approach adolescence. I hope it will continue. I have tried to maintain the balance between helping them to understand what I believe and what research bears out—that the contribution of their genetic contributors has played a very important part in who they are becoming; but that we are very much a family, and they only have one mother."[40]

My Story: How I Told Tucker

So how can we prepare children to understand and take joy in the uniqueness of their births? In my own experience, when my son was around age three and started wondering where babies came from, I kept wishing that there were a nursery rhyme I could tell him that

---

[40] Author's personal communication with Carole Lieber Wilkins.

would say it all. I thought about the story of how Superman arrived on Earth, but that was an adoption tale and didn't really fit. *Horton Hatches the Egg* by Dr. Seuss seemed closer. There was so much I loved about this story, yet so much that deeply disturbed me. The characters—the little elephant-bird who flew behind Horton and the lazy mother bird who couldn't sit still on her nest—were rife with potential misinterpretations. Would my son think his ovum donor was really the mother bird who flew off into the night after producing an egg, and later would return trying to claim him as her own? Would he see me as the nursemaid elephant and not his real mother? Was he supposed to choose me over his mother? That cascade of thoughts was not easy for me to examine. No way would those possibilities serve either of us. The "choosing" element of any story that was right for me and my son had to be a choice that was reached without ambiguity.

Finally, I decided I'd have to write my own story tailored just for Tucker, so I created a new story, complete with illustrations, to be inserted into his baby book. Tucker's baby book starts out as almost every baby book does, with a collection of newborn nursery pictures, footprints, and a hospital wrist tag. It contains a list of all the gifts he received from family and friends. Then comes the report of milestones: first smile, first time sitting up, first steps, first taste of solid food, etc. There are photos of his nursery, his crib, the garden where he crawled and played, his family members and pets, including two golden retrievers, chickens, pigs, and horses. But the next section is entitled "A Word about Me, from Mom," and that's where I placed his birth story, or I should really say his conception story, telling him all about how he came to be.

The birth story starts with an event that occurred a few years before Tucker was either born or imagined. It made such an impression on me that I had to include it in his story. It happened on a morning in 1992, shortly after David and I had bought our land in Hawaii and before we'd built our house. We were camping on our property, in the shadow of Mauna Kea, and I woke up to look out the tent flap toward a row of eucalyptus trees. I could smell their sweet lemony scent in the air, and I thought how lucky we were to be there. As I admired those magnificent trees, I saw the vision of a blonde boy-child scampering about, dancing in and out of the shadows of the trees. I woke David and told him about what I saw and how the land seemed to be speaking to me. I laughed as I reported this vision, adding that the sense of this child being a part of this place was very powerful for me, and that I had the sense that the little boy I saw was not a grandchild, and what could that mean?

Little did I know at the time how prophetic this vision would turn out to be. Our child, who would be born four years later, would come with the help of an ovum donor who came from a family with brunettes on both sides. But he would be full of blonde curls and would choose this tree-shadowed place, out of all the rest of our 36 acres, as his favorite spot to play hide-and-seek.

I began my story for Tucker with the report of this vision, calling it a "special secret" that the sky had whispered to me and that I finally came to understand in a "magical moment."

"I finally understood the secret that Mother Nature had been trying to tell me," I wrote. "I went to Daddy and told him about what I had seen as you ran about from the trees into the meadow, playing and laughing—that it was a message from your spirit-self asking me to bring you into the world.

"Mommy and Daddy set about to give you the nicest body-home for your little spirit. I found the perfect seeds to allow you to express whatever you would want to become, and then they were specially gathered and fertilized with Daddy's sperm and placed in me. One of the little seedlings you chose to enter!" (Here, I placed a photograph of the six little pre-embryo cell clusters that were growing in the laboratory right before they were transferred into my womb, one of which was destined to become Tucker.)

"As the seedling that was to be your home continued to grow and multiply its tiny cells, Mommy would talk to your spirit about what a wonderful, strong little body-home it would have. Each day I ate the best foods to help you grow. I could tell your spirit enjoyed its little body in Mommy's womb—all safe and warm. You told me how happy you were by kicking up your tiny heels and turning summersaults! I would give you massages on your little bottom and tickle your feet. We had a great system of tapping back and forth to talk to each other. Especially fun for you were the times we would go swimming. You would paddle about inside my womb as it swung gently back and forth with each of my strokes. Sometimes I would sing to you, or just whisper 'I love you' . . . to remind you that you were not alone. Soon it would be time for you to be born . . . but that is another story."

Throughout Tucker's toddler years, I read this story to him from time to time, just as we read other stories together, and he enjoyed it right along with all the other nursery tales. Then we'd shut the book and move on to another activity. I think, for me, it was a wonderful mechanism to help me accept this grand adventure. And, more importantly, Tucker relished his special story.

Tailoring Your Tale

Parents may worry a great deal about how their children will absorb the information about their conception/birth stories, but when you think about it, these ideas must seem no less fantastic to this generation of children than any other birth/conception stories have been to previous generations. Children have a wonderful way of easily accepting and expressing the fantastic.

When parents are comfortable in responding to their children's questions in a simple, straightforward way, when they convey the most important message to their ART children—that they were always planned for, long before conception occurred—then they have little cause to worry and many reasons to celebrate how their family came to be, as the following stories show us so delightfully.

Nancy: What a Five-Year-Old Tells her Best Friend

"At five, Kelly is aware that there are many ways to make a family," writes Nancy, a mom through donor ovum. "She has often told me that when she grows up and has children, she will also 'find a nice woman who will give me some eggs to use.' However, a few months ago, she announced that she's decided to adopt her children.

"Recently, while I was driving somewhere with Kelly and her best friend and classmate, Julian, I heard her telling him about her egg donor and how that egg was mixed with her daddy's sperm and then put inside my tummy for her to grow. Julian seemed a bit unclear about the concept, but he easily accepted her explanation. It was fun to be a fly on the wall for this conversation. It does make me think that Kelly has integrated this information into her sense of self, and she obviously thinks about it and wants to share this part of herself with her best friend. Who knows, perhaps she tells her teachers and others, too. This is fine with me. I want her to feel as comfortable as she can about this part of her history."

Miranda: Wizards and Magic Brews

For very young children, magic is an accepted part of life, and although some counselors may take issue with the use of fantasy in telling stories of origin, I have yet to meet an adult who recalls having identity problems as a child emanating from hearing the story of the stork or Horton hatching the egg. Magical stories are as wonderful and memorable a way as any other to introduce the miracle of science to a child. They serve to put into place the basics before moving into more detail later. Here is one way that a Minnesota mom found obviously works, as shown by her daughter, Miranda's, account of her origins:

"Mommy told me about a wonderful wizard who heard that she wanted a baby and told her he had the magic to do it. She said not every mommy needed magic, but she did. So she met with the wizard and he mixed some sperms with some eggs. Then he poured his magic brew into mommy's tummy and she hatched me out. When I'm big, I'm going to have a wizard too."

Meredith: Four Little Girls and Three Ways to Make a Family

When Meredith says that her kids believe needles, doctors, social workers, and the government are necessary to have children, she's just kidding, but she's not very far from the truth. Her four daughters entered the family in three ways. The oldest was adopted; the second was conceived in vitro, with Meredith's eggs and her husband's sperm; and the twins were conceived with donor ova. Meredith and her husband have been very open in age-appropriate ways with their children about their conception origins.

"Recently, my six-year-old adopted daughter is starting to try and make sense of the differences between her and the other kids and how we all became a family. She told me the other day that the twins, who are three, were adopted. I said, 'No, they grew in my tummy, just like you grew in your first mother's tummy, in China.' She answered that the twins were eggs in another woman first, so it was like being adopted. I was a little amazed and a bit proud at how she had reasoned this out, and told her she was right—it was similar in a way to being adopted.

"In the meantime, my middle daughter, who is five, is very competitive with her big sister and insists she has three mothers (one more than my adopted daughter) and that one of them is Chinese, too. She really wants to go one better than her big sister. But, for the most part there are really no differences—at least not yet—between them. Although I'm sure, as time goes on, each of them will have to face how they feel about how they came into the world."

Kitt: Making Eggs Out of Clay

Kitt and her husband have three children by donor ovum, five-year-old Michael, and three-year-old girl/boy twins, Jessica and Joshua. The children have heard their birth stories in simple terms many times.

"We have always been open with them," Kitt says. "We feel the information will do them good. By telling them early, even though they won't understand, at least the words will be familiar to them when they are old enough to comprehend what it all means. We hope this will help them to accept it as a normal way of conceiving children. Anyway, the twins really don't have a clue, but Michael has picked up on it. He understands that we needed another lady to help us have babies. He doesn't bring it up or ask questions, but when talking to his brother and sister about their birth, he always mentions the other lady, so we know he gets that much.

"Recently, I had Jessica with me at a baby shower and she noticed the mom-to-be's large belly and asked about it. I told her there was a baby in Aunt Mary's belly, just like she and Joshua had been in my belly. I explained that she and Joshua grew together in my belly and that's why we call them twins. Since then, she's talked a lot about it. She thinks I ate them and then threw them up. So much for understanding biology!

"When she mentioned it yet again in the car, her older brother Michael heard her and decided to clarify for the twins how babies got into bellies, using himself as an example. He told them that most mommies have eggs in their bellies and when the mommy wants a baby, an egg grows and hatches and then the doctor takes the baby out. 'But,' he said, 'our mommy didn't have eggs, so she needed to get one to take to the doctor to do an operation and put the egg in her belly. The egg grew until it was ready to hatch, and then when it hatched, the doctor took it out, and it was me!' He told Jessica and Joshua that I went back and brought two eggs to the doctor and he put them both in and then they were born the same way!

"I asked Michael where we got the eggs, and he said, 'You and daddy and that other nice lady made them!'

"'How did we make them?' I wanted to know.

"And he replied, 'Out of clay.'

"I was trying not to laugh and said, 'Why do you think it took three of us to make one egg out of clay?'

"He said, 'Well, you and Daddy had to make it together so I'd belong to both of you, and the other lady had to bring the clay!'

"That's a five-year-old's take on donor ovum and IVF. Not too bad really, if you think about it. It seems like he's really beginning to understand, even if he doesn't have the biology exactly right."

I agree that Michael is off to a great start. The role of the donor as "the other lady" is clearly separate in his mind from that of his parents. Even if someone else brings the clay, this boy knows that it is his parents who made him together.

Coleen: Sperms, Worms, and Germs

Colleen has been telling her son his birth story since she began reading to him.

"He's almost four now and he can tell the whole story," she says, "starting with how Mommy wanted a baby soooo much and used to cry and cry . . . for a long, long, long, long time. Then she went to the doctor and found out she didn't have any eggs. So a nice lady gave Mommy and Daddy an egg, and the doctor mixed it with Daddy's sperm, put it in Mommy's tummy and James grew and grew 'til he was born."

Colleen has not only told her son about his origins in an age appropriate way, but she's also provided an important context for the information—his being so very, very wanted.

"He gets sperms, germs, and worms confused," she says, "but he does talk about how he was made from Daddy's 'worms' and grew in my tummy—and he knows he was wanted very much. I believe that by treating the whole subject openly, it's no big deal. That way, later he won't be surprised or shocked. He also knows that I don't have babies easily. He's been at my doctor's appointments for the last two failed transfers. Also, as he gets more knowledgeable, the genetics of it all will be a gradual realization and no big horrifying discovery."

By bringing him along with her to her specialist appointments, Colleen is also teaching her son to appreciate that miracles don't just happen, sometimes they must be tried for again and again.

As Time Goes By

As children mature step-by-step, so does their ability to understand details about conception and birth. But their capacity to understand where babies come from may not coincide with their interest in the topic. Unless your child expresses curiosity and interest, I would not embark on any long-winded seminars. There will be plenty of occasions to open up further discussion. And, most important, you needn't feel you have to cover everything in one sitting. Children have a wonderful way of asking for more when they're ready and, from time to time, asking to have repeated what they may still be digesting.

Opportunities abound. Perhaps at the time a teacher plans to take maternity leave, or a member of the family is talking about starting a family of his or her own, your child may pop up with some comments that will open a door to exploring ideas about how babies come to be. You might explain to your child that children become part of their families in many ways, and then go on to tell your child that the way he or she arrived was really special. You might offer to tell more at this point, but if your child doesn't appear interested, just let it go.

Different issues arise at different times for children. For example, kindergarteners and first graders often find discussions about body elimination exhaustingly intriguing and will tell you endless potty jokes. But, by the time they get to be eight or nine years old, a general shift in attitude starts to appear. You might discover, as I did, that your uninhibited little boy who talks about poop and farts might also take an interest in eggs and sperm, but if you mention the sex word or penises or vaginas, he'll tell you, "That's disgusting!"

Your confidence as a parent, your willingness to be attuned to the issues that interest your children as they arise, to be a loving, active, and careful listener, will go a long way towards easing their way. Solutions may seem to crop up as you go forward in time and gain more experience living your parental role.

Recently, an unexpected opportunity arose with Tucker. I was sitting beside him at the kitchen table, looking through a clothing catalogue in which children appeared beside the adult models. There, on the front cover, was a boy a few years older than Tucker who looked the spitting image of him, golden curls, mischievous smile and all! I remarked how alike they appeared, and Tucker agreed. Then I asked him if he had any idea how it was that two people who had no relatives in common could look so much alike.

He said he didn't know, so I pulled out a sketchpad and a set of magic markers for a little science lesson. Whenever Tucker sees magic markers he knows he's in for fun, so he was interested as I wrote down three questions: How alike or unalike are we? What kind of stuff are we made of? What makes us who we are?

I drew four big circles across the top of the page to represent eggs and then filled them in with pink polka dots. I added a few dots of a different color—yellow, lime-green, orange and purple—in each circle. I told Tucker that these eggs all came from different mommies, and to notice that they were identical, except for a tiny bit of colorful stuffing in each one.

Then I suggested that we should decide whose eggs they might be and label them. Tucker chose the first to be mine, the next was our donor Kelly's, then came Tucker's brother's wife, Renee, and finally he decided the last egg would be from Aunty Edith, the mother of his best friend.

I went on to tell him that the pink polka dots represented genes, which are tiny bits of ingredients that help make a human being, passed down through all the family of man, and that only a small amount (1%) of these genes (the differently colored ones) actually were different from egg to egg, otherwise you couldn't tell the eggs apart.

Then I made other drawings for sperm, sketching pollywog shapes. I had Tucker fill them in with pink dots, putting a few different colored dots in each one. Then Tucker watched as I added a girl or a boy part to each sperm. I told him that each sperm could only have a girl ingredient or a boy ingredient, but not both. This led to a little conversation because Tucker was fascinated that it was the sperm that determined whether a baby would be a girl or a boy once it got together with the egg.

The next part of the lesson was to blend all the stuffing together to make a bundle of cells that would be an embryo. I had Tucker draw a nice dotted cluster, then we flipped the page. I intended to zoom into a single cell to show what was going on, but at that point we were interrupted. Tucker's ten-year old cousin arrived and wanted to play with him outside. So, out they went, and I closed the sketchpad and left it on the table for another day.

That evening, when both boys came in for supper, Tucker's cousin spied the catalogue cover that I had torn off and tucked into the sketchpad. He was immediately intrigued. I don't know if Tucker would have wanted to return to the science lesson, but his cousin was interested in the photo and the sketches we'd made. The combination of the two boys worked like magic to revive the discussion. We talked about what went on inside a cell's control center—I drew trees to represent chromosomes that held genes in their branches like leaves. Then I drew little "trains" that traveled up and down the trunks, depicting the RNA that would read the messages in the genes.

Next came all the good building blocks that entered the cell from the nutritious foods that an expectant mother would eat during her pregnancy. The building blocks zoomed like UFO's from a mouth to the womb, through the placenta and up the cord straight into the baby. Then I drew shapes that stood for the loving feelings and happy energy that the mom and dad shared together, and I tried to show—by sketching tiny lightning bolts—how that energy (also called hormones and neurotransmitters) flows through a pregnant woman's blood stream. The boys "saw" those little streaks of lightning going into the mom's womb-wall, through the placenta and up the cord, waking up the baby's sleepy cells. The next picture showed how the parents' feelings of love and energy helped stimulate certain brain cells to grow long arms (dendrites) that hooked up to one another and form important pathways, so that the cells within the baby's brain could begin to "talk" to each other.

The final set of drawings showed the boys a baby at a later stage of fetal development, when the brain's pathways were "wired" for loving, learning, jumping and playing, each at the right time. And yes, the fetus I was depicting was wired for blonde curls and a mischievous smile, too.

Returning to the catalogue cover, the boys and I talked a bit more about how Tucker looked so much like the young model and was so unlike him at the same time. Our conversation lasted nearly two hours, with both boys fully engaged. I know this groundwork will one day enhance both boys' understanding of genetics and preempt any simplistic misconceptions that they may have had that genes are the only things that make us unique.

But this isn't where the story involving genes and identity ends, at least not in our family. As an offshoot of my relationship with my donor, it just evolved naturally for Tucker to meet her. It was just another step of encouraged discovery in an already familiar theme. When Tucker was six, we all visited Kelly and her family on one of our frequent trips from our home in Hawaii to the mainland. We had a wonderful time. Although Tucker didn't pay much attention to any of the adults, he played easily with Kelly's son. Over the years, they've continued to exchange birthday gifts, and Tucker especially likes getting presents from Kelly's son because he always seems to know which toys are best. Kelly told me during one of our recent visits that she has developed a growing "aunty" kind of affection for my son, much the same way she has in getting to know and enjoy her little nephews over the years.

Because I believe, and I teach our son, that genetics is not an essential element for love between parents, children, or siblings, I don't think he will experience an identity problem as a result of having been created with the help of ART, even after getting to know our donor's family and understanding more about the bond Kelly and I have created between us. But if he should develop a longing to think about Kelly's children in a brotherly way in the future, then he is still likely to do so with the understanding that it is relationship that primarily makes a family. Our donor, Kelly, has four children, including one who's adopted. And if my son were to relate to them as siblings, he would probably relate to them all as such equally, because he will understand that shared genetics is only a tiny part of his bond with them. From my perspective, if he needs to think of their family as part of ours, I would happily support that. But that is because he is my son. I would do no less for him in his beliefs than I would do for either of our older children.

In Their Own Words

We now have a generation of more than 40,000 children from donor-assisted pregnancies, many already well into their teens, from whom we can learn a great deal. Most are children who have grown up in families with parents who chose to be as open as possible about their origins in an evolving, matter-of-fact, and age appropriate way.

For all teenagers, the work of establishing identity is a healthy, often stressful, part of maturing. Sorting out the ways in which they are unique, and how, at the same time, they are also a valuable part of their family is an ongoing, healthy process for adolescents. It is in no way a unique phenomenon for children of ART, although ART parents may worry that their teenagers might misinterpret or attribute difficult family issues to the circumstances of their conception.

One day, a youngster can be emulating the parent in every way, espousing the same values, and the next day, that same parent is the sworn enemy of all the teen believes in. Adolescents rocket back and forth between peer group identity and individualism, wanting so much to belong and yet rebelling at the same time. As part of that journey, it wouldn't be surprising if a teenager might test the tenacity of his or her parents' love and support by saying something as startling as: "If you don't like me the way I am, you should have thought about shopping for better eggs."

For an ART parent, this might be an opportune time to say something like: "Our disagreement isn't about eggs or your not being made out of the right stuff, any more than it would be for daddy and me, when we disagree, to say that we should trade each other in for a better made partner. If you want to talk some more about your origins with dad or me, we can certainly do that at another time, but not now. The issue right now is about us as a family and what is reasonable to expect of one another because we love each other and want to make safe and sound decisions."

This type of challenge, this "Do you really love me as I am?" kind of testing, often arises in adoptive families. So far, I haven't actually heard it reported by any ART parents, but I present the hypothetical dialogue here to assuage the fears of any ART parents who may encounter explosive adolescent emotions about their parents' assisted pregnancies. For those who wish to explore developmental attachment issues in more depth, an excellent and supportive discussion is provided in the book *Attaching in Adoption, Practical Tools for Today's Parents* by Deborah Gray.[41] I found the observations and recommendations it contains to be right on target for all teens, not just those who are adopted.

While writing this book, I asked my online group of ART mothers to run a few questions by their children. To the queries: "Is there anything you'd like me to tell prospective mothers and dads about ovum donation or donor insemination? Is there anything you think they should know beforehand?" I received a flurry of responses—all of them containing the encouragement to "Go for it!"

Fifteen-Year-Old Ken Talks about his Origins

"If you really want to have a baby and there is a way to do it, then you should go for it! I know my mom and dad are really happy they did. I know they used a donor egg to make me, and really, it's no big deal. It never gets talked about with my friends because it's not something they even think about asking. If they did, then they'd know enough about that kind of stuff that I'd be fine with telling them."

Twelve-Year-Old Tally on Understanding her Dad

"It feels like I've always known about my dad. I know he wanted me pretty badly because he looked and looked around until he could find a good sperm to make mom's egg grow. Dad doesn't mind at all. He says that I would never have been born if he hadn't looked and looked first. He says I am the best thing they ever made together and there is no one else quite like me."

---

[41] Deborah Gray, *Attaching in Adoption, Practical Tools for Today's Parents*, (Indianapolis: Perspectives Press, 2002).

Seventeen-Year-Old Kela: Forever Grateful to her Adoptive Parents

"I was adopted from Tahiti, and I know that my family of origin had some amazing people in it, like navigators, who may have even discovered the island of Hawaii where I am living now. It was my mom and dad who have taught me to take my ancestry to my heart, who shared with me my language and my proud heritage. They are hanai to me; they nurture my soul. Long after my body is gone their teachings will endure through my children. This is who I am."

Fourteen-Year-Old Ryan on the Importance of Honesty

"For as long as I can remember, it's always been just my mom and me. She's single, and I was made with the help of donor sperm. The donor was anonymous. But I know, even if I did know him, it wouldn't change my relationship with my mom—or even a future dad. That's because I think who I am, how I've developed, is one hundred percent because of how I've been raised. That's also why I believe so strongly that no kid should ever be lied to about his origins.

"My mom has always been completely up front with me. She was married when I was conceived, but the relationship did not work out, and she felt she had to leave, for both our sakes, to keep us safe. So, she's had to face a lot of difficult decisions alone—one of the biggest was choosing to take me away from the only father I might have known. Maybe if her ex-husband had wanted to get to know and love me for who I am, he would have been my dad, despite the divorce. But because I haven't had a father in my life, I've needed to sort out what parts of me are because of my upbringing and what comes from biology. Sure, I'm very interested in where I came from, but not because I want my mom's donor to be a father to me, it's more to fill in the gaps and remove the mystery that surrounds who I am. For me, the most important part of connecting with him would be to learn more about myself.

"My mom's donor was also a donor for other women. The cryobank told us that much. So I know I have at least nine half-sisters and brothers out there, and that is good to know. It makes me feel less alone. I wish there were an open policy for all donors and kids that allowed families to write or exchange pictures—or even meet each other, if everyone were comfortable. That would be my ideal. I'd like just to see if Mom's donor or my half-siblings and I share some of our looks—that would be so special. My mom and I started a donor registry as a way of helping kids of donor assisted pregnancies to meet and share their common bonds, if they choose to make a connection."

The Donor Sibling Registry that Ryan and his mother created began as a Yahoo group in September, 2000 and has since grown to a full web data base for hundreds of clinics and cryobanks all over the world. More than 4000 families and individuals have registered, and the site has facilitated almost 800 half-sibling matches at this time, averaging about 15 matches a month.

Ryan knows that his mother and the other families who received sperm from the same donor were all advised never to tell anyone that they used donor assistance—a policy that has created a lot of frustration for him, as it has for many other ART families. It's painful for Ryan to accept that his half siblings may never know that there are others in the world related to them, whom they might wish to know, if given the chance.

Someday, perhaps, these individuals may learn that their DNA has a story to tell, different from what they had assumed. Fate may take a hand in revealing the truth. Circumstances may lead to discovery. But until then, Ryan and others like him must live with the consequences of poor counseling and the fallout from an attitude that secrecy is somehow beneficial when it absolutely is not, as the experience of so many ART families have shown, including my own.

"No kid should ever be lied to about his origins," Ryan reminds us. Then he goes on to say, "I mean it. And to me, not telling the whole story is lying."

I couldn't agree more.

When the adopted Chinese daughter of a professional friend of mine heard that I was writing a book for ART parents, she contacted me and offered the following autobiographical essay, which she felt might help ART parents. It won first prize in a state writing contest.

The Return

By Theresa Tanner

Once there was a girl named Jayme. She was 13-years-old, had ebony hair, black eyes and a magnificent smile. After dinner, Jayme talked to her parents about her past and her adoption. Her face looked unhappy and sad. She wanted to go to China to find her parents, but how? Jayme started to pack her clothes and some money. Her parents loved Jayme very much, so they packed some clothes too. They rode to the airport and bought three tickets.

When Jayme got off the plane in China she noticed that everyone had ebony hair and black eyes. Jayme thought this was a good sign. Of course she could find her parents. Jayme and her parents went to her orphanage and asked about her Chinese parents. The staff still had a paper her mother had written in Chinese: "Please take care of my child for me. We are poor and we cannot provide her good clothes or food to eat." When Jayme and her family went to find Jayme's Chinese mother there was no one living anymore in the old apartment. The people next door said they had moved years ago and didn't know where they had moved to. Jayme was heartbroken. *Maybe my mom did the right thing for me. She probably wanted to protect me from suffering. Perhaps I came to China to discover what China is all about. I discovered my Chinese language and where I was born.* Jayme said, "Mom and Dad, I just wanted to see what China looked like. Perhaps I cannot have what I wanted, but I can have the both of you." All three of them hugged each other and went out for Chinese food.

In her story, Theresa shows us through Jayme that she was able to accept what could be known about her origins and, at the same time, identify with her adopted family and move on. This kind of maturity does not come by accident. As children get older, if they are comfortable in the embrace of their parents' love, they will bring forth important questions and insecurities. What a wonderful family Theresa has, responding so readily to her expressed need to find out more about herself.

Letting Love Multiply

So here we are, having come full circle through the ART experience as told by parents who've taken the daunting journey, the children who've reached life against the odds, and those who've helped make the journey possible.

As I've recounted the experiences of those who have chosen parenthood as the cherished top priority in their lives, I've been struck by how little society rewards those efforts. The struggle of these individuals to create and nurture children goes well beyond the desire to produce a new generation in one's own image, or to have a living repository for one's inheritance. It is about the sense of completion that comes from the conscious commitment to be responsible for the well being of another. It is the wisdom that comes from the ashes of loss, translated into new life.

Parents such as these set an example for all of us about the hard work of love. It is my hope that in this collection of reflections, including my own, this richly deserving group of individuals can find support and understanding that goes beyond naïve optimism and that will help them in their own journey and in the clearing of an easier path for those who follow. Being parents in today's world is not an easy task for anyone; my highest respect goes out to all of them, and I wish them all the best.

Afterword

For those who work in the field of reproductive endocrinology and infertility, there is homework to be done and lessons to be learned.

As physicians and therapists, our primary ethical responsibility is to address the psyche of our patients before picking up the tools of our trade to mend their bodies. We have marched forward with technology, creating family building options that have major emotional implications for our patients who are living in an unprepared, reactionary society. The professional literature describing ART must move beyond the language of adoption in explaining the miracle of technology that has permitted the building of families through ART. Therapists who counsel patients struggling with issues relating to ART need to understand what is unique about ART and to listen carefully to the stories of these courageous individuals. There is great wisdom and compassion in their stories.

We as professionals must respect and honor the values and wishes of our patients as they make their choices among the options now available to them in starting a family, and as they consider their options regarding disclosure of private information to their children. But we must also be clear in our own minds about what it means to be a parent and about the rights of children to be treated with openness, honesty, and love as they discover who they are and where they came from. If we are not clear about these issues, how can we expect our patients to be clear about them? How can we expect our patients to raise children who will feel accepted and loved?

Appendix I

Basic Facts about Infertility

For some women, pregnancy is so simple and easy—nature takes its course and, ready or not, three things happen:

1. Ovulation—release of the egg
2. Fertilization—union of sperm and egg
3. Implantation—burrowing of embryo into the lining of the uterus.

When this process gets interrupted at any step along the way, there will be trouble. Today, nearly six million couples in America are affected by infertility, technically defined as the inability to conceive after one year of unprotected intercourse. From this group, nearly two million couples will need the help of a fertility specialist. Experts disagree about the exact percentages, but roughly a little less than half of the time, the problem is due to the man's reproductive system. About a third of the time, the problem lies with the woman. And the remaining cases may be a combined problem or simply unexplained. This is why it's important that both partners get a medical work up.

Common Causes of Female Infertility

- *Endometriosis.* Normally, the glandular and stromal endometrial cells that make up the lining of the uterus, and that grow during the menstrual cycle under the influence of estrogen and progesterone, are found only in the uterus. However, sometimes endometrial cells grow outside of the uterus and cause scarring, pain, and heavy bleeding. This condition, called endometriosis, can damage the fallopian tubes and ovaries and is a common cause of infertility.
- *Blockage of fallopian tubes.* This is a condition typically caused by scar tissue from prior pelvic infections or surgeries.
- *Failure to ovulate.* This problem has many causes. A woman receives her full supply of oocytes (eggs) during her development as a fetus. At the time of her birth, she has about one to two million. By puberty, a healthy young girl will have about 300,000 eggs remaining, each tucked into its own tiny pocket of cells (follicle) within the ovary, programmed to respond to hormonal fluctuations. The adult female body is designed to allow only one egg to mature and be released each month. Any other eggs that may have started to mature during the same cycle will soon degenerate as the first follicle becomes dominant and eventually releases the egg it carries (ovulation). Throughout the reproductive years, usually between the ages of 13 and 45, a woman will ovulate approximately 400 times. During the later years, her sensitivity to hormone cycling will diminish, and the release of eggs will become irregular. Eventually, her ovulation and menses will stop altogether. She has then reached menopause.

  In addition to normal menopause, failure to ovulate can be due to:

  - Ovaries that arrested in their growth during fetal development.
  - Failure of the brain during puberty to produce the hormones that trigger maturation of the

reproductive system so that ovulation and menstrual cycling occurs.
- If a woman has too few eggs, her supply will be exhausted in her 20s or 30s, a condition called premature ovarian failure. In some cases this can happen before puberty is reached.
- Eggs becoming trapped within follicles.
- An imbalance of hormones preventing a single follicle from becoming dominant, a condition called polycystic ovary syndrome.

- *Luteal phase problem.* When an inadequate amount of progesterone is released during the second phase of the menstrual cycle, the uterine lining will not undergo the changes required for an embryo to properly embed and grow.
- *Uterine problems.* Fibroids or other uterine growths can interrupt implantation. Anomalies in the shape of the uterus, or the presence of an intrauterine septum, can prevent the embryo from finding an ideal place to imbed or grow.
- *Mucous problems.* Mucous at the entrance to the cervix may be too thick for the sperm to penetrate, or it may be toxic to sperm.
- *Genetic problems.* When a developing pre-embryo has inherited genetic problems, the woman's body may spontaneously abort it.
- *Advanced age.* Germ cells of older women may still have the right number of chromosomes, but in forming the zygote at conception, the cytoplasm cannot direct the chromosomes to properly line up for subdivision, and genetic information gets either duplicated or lost.

Common Causes of Male Infertility

- *Low sperm count.* There are a number of causes of low or abnormal sperm count. If the condition is due to toxins or chemicals, the sperm count may return to normal after a few months. If the condition is due to radiation therapy or certain viral infections, the sperm count may never return to normal. If there are still some healthy sperm present, a single sperm may be all that is necessary for fertilization. To enable fertilization by a single viable sperm, intracytoplasmic sperm injection (ICSI) will be required. If no normal sperm are found, a sperm donor will be needed.

- *Sperm that are weak swimmers.* Sperm that are weak swimmers may not reach the egg or may reach the egg but fail to penetrate the egg wall. Sometimes ICSI can be used to overcome this problem. Using this laboratory procedure, an REI specialist can insert a single sperm into an egg.
- *Varicoceles.* These are abnormally dilated veins along the spermatic cord that cause temperature changes in the testicles, affecting sperm development and survival. Varicoceles can often be surgically repaired or embolized (a procedure to block off the dilated veins), but those procedures do not always result in healthy sperm.
- *Damaged sperm ducts.* These may be due to scarring associated with sexually transmitted diseases (STDs) or a prior vasectomy. Sometimes the ducts can be reconnected following vasectomy, but the antibodies built up during the time of obstruction can remain a problem.
- *Hormonal deficiency.* If a male has a hormonal deficiency so that sperm can't be produced or cannot properly mature, replacement of the missing hormones may help. A biopsy of the testis may be necessary to help determine the severity of the problem.
- *Testicular failure.* This can be caused by tumors, drugs, trauma, viral infections (e.g., mumps), some sexually transmitted diseases (STDs), or a prior vasectomy. When sperm are blocked within the testis for long periods of time (as with vasectomy), the male forms antibodies to his own sperm that interfere with their transport and function. Sometimes these sperm can be

medically treated in a laboratory and directly injected into the egg (ICSI).
- *Sperm antibodies.* Antibodies produced by a female partner can incapacitate and kill sperm. IUI (intrauterine insemination) allows the sperm to bypass hostile cervical mucus, or IVF (in vitro fertilization) can be performed in the laboratory using ICSI with sperm that have been previously washed to remove antibodies.

Appendix II

What To Expect: Common Tests and Procedures

Most women who are having difficulty getting pregnant will work with their Ob/Gyn for the initial testing and evaluation that will be needed to identify the reason or reasons for the difficulty. Their Ob/Gyn will follow accepted work-up protocols and order some basic tests. The results of these tests may lead to an early resolution of the infertility problem at relatively modest cost. Or they may suggest the need for more complex, and more expensive, procedures and testing that are best done by a reproductive endocrinology and infertility (REI) specialist.

If you need the help of an REI specialist, your Ob/Gyn can make a referral, or you can contact a specialist organization such as the Society for Assisted Reproductive Technology (SART) in order to locate a clinic near to you. SART's website address is *http://sart.org/home.html*. Understand that not all SART clinics are run by board certified REI specialists. So, there is one further step I would recommend before selecting a clinic, and that is to check whether the clinic's REI specialist is a board certified member of the Society for Reproductive Endocrinology and Infertility (SREI). If you contact SREI at their website *http://www.socrei.org/*, you can enter the name of your SART clinic physician to see if he or she has taken the specialty boards.

Having this certification process is important because it means that your physician will have completed an additional three to four years training in infertility after his or her basic residency experience.

Health history. Be prepared to answer questions about your childhood illnesses, surgeries, and medications for past treatments or current conditions. You'll also be asked about your prior reproductive history—births, miscarriages, abortions or neonatal deaths—and your sexual history, including any exposure to sexually transmitted diseases. Your Ob/Gyn will need to know if you have a family history of birth defects, problems perhaps diagnosed later in life such as kidney or neurological diseases, mental retardation, or infertility in other family members, or if either you or your partner has been exposed to hazardous substances.

Ovarian reserve testing. Follicle Stimulating Hormone (FSH) and Estradiol levels will be drawn on day 3 of your cycle, or possibly a Clomid challenge test will be given to assess ovarian function.

Physical exam. After a careful history is obtained, you'll be given a complete physical exam, including examination of the pelvic organs. In addition to palpation of the vagina, cervix, uterus, fallopian tubes, ovaries, and rectum, cervical cultures and a pap smear will be taken.

Sperm analysis. Your Ob/Gyn may order laboratory tests of your partner's urine, semen, and blood, including a measurement of serum testosterone level. If abnormalities are found, your partner may be referred to an andrologist, a specialist trained to deal with all aspects of male infertility. If the semen analysis is repeatedly abnormal—i.e., if there are too few sperm or the movement of the sperm is abnormal—ICSI (intracytoplasmic sperm injection) may help to successfully fertilize the ovum.

Post-coital test. You may be asked to visit your Ob/Gyn's office within a few hours after intercourse so that a post coital test can be performed. This test, which is being used less and less often, involves the taking of a sample of cervical mucous with a swab and the examination of the sample under a microscope to assess the quality of cervical mucous (it should be abundant, watery, and "stringy," with a normal pH and ferning pattern noted) and to see if there are viable sperm that are normal in appearance and that show good motility. Sometimes the sperm appear normal but are few in number, are clumped together, or show poor motility and are only shaking in place. Such findings may suggest the presence of anti-sperm antibodies, from either the male or female, that are hostile to sperm. If no sperm are found, or if the sperm have an abnormal appearance, a thorough assessment of the male partner will usually be done.

Testing for ovulation. Common tests for ovulation include temperature charting and simple urine and/or blood hormone tests. Examination of cervical mucous is also helpful. If a woman isn't ovulating, her cervical secretions will not show the characteristic pre-ovulation ferning pattern under the microscope, nor will they show the subsequent post-ovulation loss of this pattern, something that occurs when progesterone is produced after the egg has left the follicle.

If a woman is not ovulating, she can be given medications to induce release of an egg. This treatment is known as ovarian stimulation or hormonal manipulation, and it can lead, at times, to multiple ovulation, which may mean triplets, quadruplets, or even more babies!

Some studies suggest that fertility drugs increase the risk of ovarian cancer, but these results are controversial, not only because the studies were so small, but also because we don't know if the increased risk of cancer is secondary to the infertility state or the treatment. Currently, the medical establishment recommends that ovulation-inducing medications not be used for more than six months. Since time is of the essence, it's critical that this treatment be accompanied by adequate monitoring, including an ultrasound series to closely observe the growth and number of follicles being stimulated, and additional drug therapy to control the precise timing of ovulation.

Ultrasound. Your Ob/Gyn may perform or order an ultrasound evaluation of the uterus to assess the thickness of the uterine lining or to look for anomalies or irregularities either in the uterine wall or protruding into the uterine cavity. An ultrasound machine is typically used in an office setting and does not require special anesthesia. This machine uses high frequency sound waves sent from a probe that is placed high in the vagina. These sound waves produce a detailed image on the viewing screen not only of the contents of the uterine cavity but also of various pelvic structures as the waves bounce off of these structures. This allows the internal as well as pelvic anatomy to be seen without having to resort to surgery. Ultrasound information can help determine the next steps in treatment.

Saline infusion sonohysterography (SIS). Ultrasound evaluation of the internal anatomy of the uterus can be enhanced by injecting salt solution into the uterine cavity through a small tube and then looking at the uterine cavity by intravaginal ultrasound probe.

Artificial insemination (AI). AI includes an array of procedures, some of which have been in use for more than 50 years, to help couples overcome hostile or insufficient cervical mucous, structural abnormalities of the reproductive organs, or unexplained infertility. An intended father's fresh sperm, or a donor's frozen sperm, can be directed into the cervix (intracervical insemination or ICI), or washed sperm without seminal fluid can be introduced directly into the uterus (intrauterine insemination or IUI), bypassing the cervix.

As a general rule, I recommend that women undergo no more than three cycles of ICI/IUI treatments before seeking a more extensive evaluation from a fertility expert. The success rate of IUI for women under age forty, with no evidence of organic pelvic disease, is around 10% to 15% per cycle.[42] For women over forty, the success rates are not as good. For these women, and for younger women whose ovaries need to be stimulated, moving to IVF might be preferable.

The foregoing tests and procedures are more or less routine. If these do not lead to identification and resolution of the problem, other more complex and expensive tests and procedures may be required. These include:

---

[42] G. Sher, MD, V.M. Davis, RN, MN., and J. Stoess, MA, *In Vitro Fertilization, the A.R.T. of Making Babies*, (New York: Facts on File, Inc., 1995) 146-149.

Saline hysterogram. A thin tube containing an optical scope and a passageway for tiny surgical instruments (hysteroscope) is inserted through the cervix while injecting salt solution into the uterine cavity to enhance the ability to diagnose intracavitary lesions. Sometimes polyps, sub-mucous fibroids, and other obstructions such as an internal septum (dividing wall) or intrauterine adhesions can be removed under mild sedation in the office without more extensive surgery. If more extensive surgery is anticipated, the doctor usually recommends performing the hysteroscopic procedure in an operating room under heavy sedation or general anesthesia.

Hysterosalpingogram (HSG). While using X-ray guidance for intermittent viewing, the doctor inserts dye through the cervix and into the uterine cavity through a tiny tube attached to a syringe, making the outline of the cavity of the uterus visible on a screen. If the fallopian tubes are open, the dye will be seen streaming out of the ends. Should the tubes be blocked, the procedure could become quite painful if an attempt is made to open the ends of the tubes by applying increased pressure through the syringe. Since the degree of blockage can't be known in advance, it might be preferable to ask for pain medication before the start of the procedure and to bring someone to the hospital or doctor's office to drive you home. Most women experience only mild, transient cramping during a hysterosalpingogram, but if the tubes are blocked, severe cramping could linger after the procedure. It never hurts to be pre-medicated and prepared. Many women with blocked tubes will find themselves pregnant a few months after this procedure because the pressure of the fluid can be sufficient to open up the tubes. If a major blockage is found, surgery or IVF is usually recommended.

Laparoscopy. Under anesthesia, a thin tube containing an optical scope with laser or cautery attachment is inserted into the abdomen through the navel to examine the pelvic structures, tubes, and ovaries. During the procedure, scar tissue and irritating endometrial cell implants can be excised with scissors or vaporized or burned away with the laser or cautery attachment. But if there is extensive scarring in the pelvis, or if the ovaries are involved with large endometriomas (blood-filled cysts), an open operation with a larger incision into the abdominal wall may be necessary.

Reconnecting fallopian tubes. An Ob/Gyn or REI specialist who is an expert micro-surgeon can also reconnect tubes previously severed by ligation, or re-open the tubal fimbria (fronds at the end of the fallopian tubes that pick up the egg) that may have been closed by scar tissue due to previous infection. This surgery is delicate, however, and its success will depend on the extent of initial tubal damage and the expertise of the surgeon. Careful monitoring is necessary after the procedure because of the possibility of an ectopic (tubal) pregnancy (implantation of the embryo in the repaired tube).

Appendix III

Ethics and Embryos

ART isn't just physically and emotionally challenging. It also raises a host of ethical issues or questions. Here are some of the ones that have challenged my thinking.

Is Parenthood a Person's Right?

Do people who are infertile have a right to attempt to have a child? I say absolutely yes. Couples suffering from infertility have a medical condition that limits their ability to live their lives to their fullest. Their inability to have children can create suffering as real as that resulting from any other malady. For one thing, infertility causes enormous stress, which is one of the causes of heart disease, stroke, cancer, and decreased immune system function. What's more, stress can further complicate infertility by producing an abnormal release of hormones from the brain, blocking or interfering with the release of ova. The bottom line is that infertility is a medical condition that affects one's quality of life and may well be associated with the development of other significant health risks. And everyone has a right to treatment for his or her medical conditions.

The United Nations, too, has recognized that founding a family is a basic human right. Article 16 of the United Nations Declaration of Human Rights, written in 1948, states: *"Men and women of full age, without any limitation due to race, nationality or religion, have the right to marry and found a family."* Note that it doesn't say that the right to found a family belongs only to people who happen to be fertile.

Are Doctors Obliged to Help the Infertile?

Yes. The Hippocratic Oath states clearly that the physician's duty is to apply all available skill and science to help a patient attain health. The modern version of the Hippocratic Oath says, in part: *"I will apply, for the benefit of the sick, all measures which are required, avoiding those twin traps of over treatment and therapeutic nihilism . . . I will respect the privacy of my patients, for their problems are not disclosed to me that the world may know. . . . I will remember that I do not treat a fever chart, a cancerous growth, but a sick human being, whose illness may affect the person's family and economic stability. My responsibility includes these related problems, if I am to care adequately for the sick."*[43]

Is IVF Ethically or Morally Wrong?

Some ethicists have argued that IVF/ART is wrong because it manipulates human life by creating it in the laboratory in the form of a zygote (a fertilized egg cell before it starts to divide) without insuring that every zygote is given an opportunity to grow into a child. These critics point out that some zygotes mature into embryos that are frozen and are never transferred to the mother's womb, while others mature into embryos that are transferred and grow for several weeks, only to be denied an opportunity for birth as a result of selective reduction. They argue, in effect, that IVF/ART fails to honor the sanctity of the zygote or embryo and its presumed right to life. Some also regard IVF/ART as "man playing God" and intervening inappropriately into a natural process.

---

[43] Written in 1964 by Louis Lasagna, Academic Dean of the School of Medicine at Tufts University, and used in many medical schools today.

Issues relating to the ethics of IVF/ART are linked to the fundamental questions: What is human life, and when does it begin? Are human interventions that prevent or interfere with the growth of new human life always wrong? Everyone must answer these questions for him- or herself. My own comfort with the ethics of IVF/ART is shaped by three factors:

1. my understanding of how embryos develop,
2. my belief that important ethical issues involve a balancing of interests or values and are rarely, if ever, black-and-white matters of right and wrong, and
3. the fact that all children born via IVF/ART result from a purposeful commitment by loving parents and the efforts of skilled professionals applied specifically and exclusively to help those parents create life.

All embryos start as a single-celled organism called a zygote, an ovum to which the chromosomes from a sperm have been added. Within a day of fertilization, the zygote divides into two identical cells, then four, then eight, etc. This is the preembryo[44] or morula stage of development, and all cells during this stage are undifferentiated or identical. Some are destined to become placenta, and some will become embryo tissue, but it is impossible to say which will be which. Cell differentiation into different tissue types does not begin until after the morula has reached 30 to 40 cells in size. This occurs by the end of the first week, but it takes several more days before the differentiated cells have migrated to the sites where they will eventually organize themselves into different organs and systems. These organs and systems, including in particular

---

[44] The term "preembryo" is objectionable to some writers who regard it as a term adopted for political reasons by "pro-choice" advocates to support their position on abortion and by those who support embryonic stem cell and related research. See, e.g., C.W. Kischer, *The Big Lie in Human Embryology: The Case of the Preembryo,* (Kochi, Japan: Lifeissues.net, 2004); http://www.lifeissues.net/writers/kisc/kisc_11bigliepreembryo.html.

the central nervous system, do not begin to show primitive function for several more weeks.[45] If all goes well, an embryo that implants in the uterus of a healthy woman will continue to grow into a fetus that will deliver normally at approximately 40 weeks gestation, but that will become "viable," i.e., able to survive, with medical assistance, outside the uterus, sometime around 23 weeks gestation.

There are two aspects of this developmental history of the embryo that are significant to me in thinking about the ethics or morality of IVF/ART. First, there is the fact that all critical decisions that determine which embryos will be transferred and given every chance to grow occur early in embryo development, long before embryos have the neurological capacity for sentience or awareness.[46] (Capacity for awareness is the basis on which many people make value judgments about, and shape their behavior toward, different life forms. And capacity for self-awareness is what many believe distinguishes humans from other higher order species.)

Second, for all our scientific advances, there is still a great deal we do not know, and cannot predict, about embryo development. Many embryos that get their start in vivo, through intercourse, and that appear to be developing normally, will spontaneously abort, passing out undetected at or around the time of menses, or stop growing and be resorbed into the mother. Such may well be nature's way of preventing the birth of a child with genetic anomalies or other

---

[45] Electrical activity in the central nervous system is discernible by electro-encephalograph (EEG) at about 40 days gestation.

[46] Embryologist Clifford Grobstein maintains that "internal conscious awareness does not occur until at least eight weeks gestation." C. Grobstien, "The Status and Uses of Early Human Developmental Stages," *Ethical Issues in Research*, D. Cheney ed. (Maryland: The University Publishing Group, Inc., 1993).For an excellent discussion of the development of the human neurological system, see A. Sheibel, *Embryological Development of the Human Brain,* (Seattle, Washington: New Horizons for Learning, 2002), available on the Internet at www.newhorizons.org/neuro/sheibel.htm.

problems. Similarly, embryos conceived in vitro that appear to be developing normally both before and after transfer to the mother may spontaneously abort or stop growing and be resorbed. The decisions that a woman undergoing IVF makes with her REI specialist regarding the number of embryos to transfer are decisions made to maximize the chance that a healthy new life can be sustained. In a sense, these decisions mimic the decisions that nature makes.

Those who believe that life begins at conception and that an embryo, or even a zygote, is a human being who should be accorded the full status and all the rights of a viable fetus or newborn will likely find the foregoing discussion irrelevant. They view the development of a fetus from zygote to birth as a continuum, and they regard as politically motivated all descriptions of embryo development in terms of stages or functional milestones. They argue that any medical procedure that results in the creation of life without allowing such life to grow into a child is wrong. I agree that embryonic development is a continuum, and I don't take issue with the view that human life begins at conception. I just don't feel that IVF/ART is incompatible with such views. This is where a balancing of interests or values comes into play.

All life is precious, but most of us do not regard or treat all life in the same manner. We consume plant species in order that we may live, and those of us who are not vegetarian also consume many animal species. We make value judgments and engage in a balancing of interests when we sacrifice animals for medical research. Most of us are able to accept the idea that individual animals will be killed, so long as their deaths serve research that may lead to a cure for diseases that cause human suffering.

This balancing of interests also occurs when difficult decisions are made affecting the survival of human life. The laws of all states now allow hospitals and physicians to honor advance health care directives or "living wills" from individuals who do not want so-called "heroic" measures taken to prolong their lives under certain circumstances. These individuals have, in effect, weighed in advance their interest in having their last hours or days of life be dignified and unsupported by hospital-based medical technology against their interest in having their lives prolonged without regard to the quality of the prolonged life.

Other life or death decisions that involve assigning different relative values to human life, although often agonizing, are also made from time to time, and with the blessing of our judicial system. For example, in time of war, commanders in the field must frequently make decisions they know will result in the death of the men under their command. They make these decisions reluctantly, but with the understanding that they are justified and that they will result in the saving of other lives. Our criminal laws recognize self defense or defense of another as full justification for the taking of a life. What mother, seeing her child attacked and in imminent danger of death would not willfully take the life of the attacker? And those who support the death penalty are also impliedly endorsing a diminished status view of the person to be executed.

These situations all require a weighing of interests and often an assigning of greater or lesser status to some human lives relative to others. Nowhere is this more evident than in the U.S. Supreme Court's 1973 *Roe v. Wade* decision, which held that a woman's right to privacy encompasses the right to make decisions about her own child bearing, including a qualified right to have an abortion. It also recognized that states have a legitimate interest in protecting what it described as the "prenatal life,"[47] the "potential human life,"[48] or the "potentiality of human life"[49] that the fetus represents.[50] This interest increases as the fetus matures, and when the fetus reaches viability at approximately the end of the second trimester, the state's interest becomes "compelling"[51] such that the state can regulate and even

---

[47] *Roe v. Wade*, 410 U.S. 113, 155 (1973).
[48] Ibid. 159.
[49] Ibid. 162-164.
[50] The Court held that "the word 'person' as used in the Fourteenth Amendment does not include the unborn." Ibid. 158. It also declined to "resolve the difficult question of when life begins." Ibid. 159.
[51] Ibid. 163

prohibit abortion altogether. However, the Court also held that even during the third trimester, a woman's right to an abortion trumps the state's rights to protect the life of the fetus when an abortion is "necessary, in appropriate medical judgment, for the preservation of the life or health of the [woman]."[52]

Roe v. Wade is, of course, anathema to pro-life advocates. They argue, as did the state of Texas in *Roe*, that a fetus is a person and entitled to the Constitutional rights of a person from conception. But, as the Court in *Roe* noted, "when Texas urges that a fetus in entitled to Fourteenth Amendment protection as a person, it faces a dilemma. Neither in Texas nor in any other state are all abortions prohibited.... [A]n exception always exists... for an abortion procured or attempted by medical advice for the purpose of saving the life of the mother.... But if the fetus is a person who is not to be deprived of life without due process of law, and if the mother's condition is the sole determinant, does not the Texas exception appear to be out of line with the Amendment's command?"[53]

It should be clear from the foregoing examples, and from both the Court's holding in *Roe v. Wade* and the "dilemma" faced by Texas and other states with similar criminal anti-abortion laws, that the complex world in which we live presents us with many instances where we have to make life or death decisions by engaging in a balancing of interests. It is simply not possible to determine, based on science or ethics or religion, when human life begins and then have that determination alone dictate what acts or omissions are acceptable with respect to that life.[54]

---

[52] Ibid. 164
[53] Ibid. 157, FN 54.
[54] The Ethics Committee of the American Society for Reproductive Medicine has taken the position that a human embryo is a "potential human being worthy of special respect," but "not entitled to the same rights as persons." Ethics Committee of the American Society for Reproductive Medicine, "Donating Spare Embryos for Embryonic Stem Cell Research," *Fertility and Sterility*, Vol. 78, No. 5, November 2002, 958.

This brings me to the third reason I am comfortable with the ethics of IVF/ART: the motivation of those seeking IVF/ART and those performing the procedures. As I noted above, children born via IVF/ART are a unique and very special group because *all* such children result from a purposeful commitment by loving parents, and from the efforts of skilled professionals applied specifically and exclusively to help those parents create life. I believe that this circumstance is relevant and important when considering the fact that IVF usually results in the creation of embryos that are frozen and not transferred and sometimes involves selective reduction in order to maximize a woman's chances of successfully carrying and delivering a healthy child while minimizing the risks to her health (and to the health of the child or children she carries to term) from higher order pregnancies.

While I fully support the rights of women outlined and defended in the *Roe v. Wade* decision, there are aspects of the decision that trouble me, and I confess I am disturbed by the fact that the precious freedom of choice guaranteed by *Roe* seems to me to be abused on occasion. For example, I have had colleagues with patients who made no efforts at contraception and had repeated unwanted pregnancies that they then sought to have terminated in the first or second trimester, using abortion as a form of birth control. This troubles me because they are acting in a way that suggests they attach less importance to the life growing within them than they do to their convenience or lifestyle. In other words, their motives in interrupting the continuum of fetal development within them seem to me to be insubstantial. By contrast, the motives of the couple that seeks IVF are, to my way of thinking, ethically unassailable. They are seeking to create life, and the efforts and sacrifices they are making in pursuit of this goal are the very essence of love.[55] And the technology applied

---

[55] I share Dr. M. Scott Peck's view that love is far more than a feeling or sentiment. It's true expression requires the purposeful or willful expenditure of effort in pursuit of a worthwhile end. See Peck, 81. (Love is "the will to extend one's self for the purpose of nurturing one's own or another's personal growth.")

in support of the effort by the REI specialist, the embryologist, and the other staff at the REI clinic is all directed toward the same end, not toward the creation of embryos for research purposes.

To summarize, the fact that IVF/ART may involve the creation of some embryos that are frozen and not transferred, or that are sacrificed through selective reduction, is, to me, ethically and morally acceptable given the early stage of embryo development at which the key events occur, the nature of the competing interests involved, and the context within which the interests are weighed, including, in particular, the motives of both the couples and the medical professionals making the decisions.

What about the Selecting of Some Embryos for Transfer while Rejecting Others?

Part of the IVF process involves selecting embryos that are more likely than others to result in a viable pregnancy. Based on the reasoning I have outlined above, I have concluded that this process doesn't capriciously and unethically select one human being over another for life or death. The process by which embryos are graded and selected for fresh transfer is based solely on the likelihood they will survive the transfer process and successfully implant in the uterus. Of the remaining embryos, only those likely to survive the freezing and thawing will be saved. This selection process mimics what we observe in nature. The fittest are the ones most likely to survive.

Is there a Risk of People Trying for "Designer Babies?"

I don't like the phrase "designer babies," although I hear it or read it more and more. Most of us would agree that selecting embryos most likely to result in a pregnancy and birth of a baby makes sense. But some are uncomfortable about selecting donors for things like intelligence, athleticism, or attractiveness. They worry that this sort of selection process is a form of eugenics. I don't agree. Don't we select a life partner—the potential co-parent of our children—based on his or her desirable traits? And so it should be for the selection of donors.

Who is the "Real Parent" of an IVF Child?

Science can now separate out the genetic, gestational, and nurturing components of parenthood. It is now possible for two people to produce a child with whom they will never have a moment's contact. As donors of sperm and ova that will be joined in vitro to create an embryo that will be carried, delivered, and raised by someone else, they can be nothing more than providers of bits of genetic information. How can they be called "parents" under such circumstances? As I see it, the essence of "parenting" is the nurturing and raising of a child. The person that nurtures and protects and loves the child is that child's parent. I do not like the terms "genetic mother," "genetic father," or "genetic parent." The woman who provides an egg so that another woman can bear and raise a child is that child's "ovum donor" or "egg donor" or even a "genetic donor" or a "genetic contributor," but not a "parent" of any kind. To try to describe the roles of donors, or even gestational carriers, by adding different modifiers to the words "mother," "father," or "parent" is counterproductive in my opinion. I discuss this in greater detail in Chapters 4 and 5.

Is the Compensation of Donors Unethical?

Most of us in the baby boomer generation had male college classmates or other male friends who donated sperm anonymously to a sperm bank to earn a little extra money. The practice of sperm donation for money continues today, with payments to donors in the range of $50 to $80 per donation.

Ovum donation began in the early 1980s. The earliest donors were friends or relatives of the ova recipients and made the donations without compensation, but the practice of compensating ovum donors soon followed, in part to offset the donors' travel expenses, lost time from work, etc., and in part to encourage women to donate.

In the mid 1980s, ovum donors were paid about $250 per cycle. By the 1990s, compensation amounts had risen to the $1,000 to $2,000 range, and by 2000 compensation had reached $3,000 to $5,000. As of January 2005, one ovum donation program that advertised itself on the Internet as "the oldest and largest program in the world,"[56] was quoting fees of $5,000 to $15,000, with "additional compensation . . . offered to those donors who have earned a postgraduate degree [or] have a unique skill, characteristic, or trait . . . ."[57] There have been reports of ovum donation programs that advertise for donors from Ivy League colleges, offering fees of $35,000 to $50,000,[58] and at least one website solicits ova from models and other women who are "beautiful, healthy, intelligent and between 18-32 yrs. old,"[59] offering to auction such ova to recipients willing to pay up to $150,000.[60]

Few people are comfortable with the idea of self-styled "beautiful people" auctioning their ova for such sums, or with the idea of huge premiums being paid for ova from highly educated or talented donors. But most ovum donations in the United States are handled by donor programs affiliated with reputable REI clinics, and most such programs compensate donors a fixed fee of $5,000 or less, with all donors to a particular program receiving the same fee. Moreover,

---

[56] Egg Donation, Inc., http://www.eggdonor.com/?section=donor&page=fincomp.

[57] Ibid.

[58] See K. Lopez, "Eggheads, Young Women in Need of Cash are Increasingly Deciding to Sell their Bodies," *National Review* 1 Sept. 1998: 50(16):26; http://www.nationalreview.com/lopez/lopez200403260930.asp.

[59] http://www.ronsangels.com/index2.html.

[60] This website is run by a fashion photographer. It is not clear whether the site really acts as a go-between for ovum donors and recipients or whether it is primarily a mechanism for finding models for different genres of photography.

most programs clearly describe the fee as compensation for travel time, time lost from work waiting for retrieval and during the retrieval itself, risks and discomfort, side effects from medication, etc. Compensation is not described as a payment for ova as if they were commodities, and it does not depend on the number of ova retrieved or the number of successful pregnancies achieved from donated ova.

The Ethics Committee of the American Society for Reproductive Medicine issued a report in 2000 that discusses the ethics of compensating ovum donors and concludes that such compensation "may be defended on ethical grounds,"[61] provided payments are "fair and not so substantial that they become undue inducements that will lead donors to discount risks. Monetary compensation should reflect the time, inconvenience, and physical and emotional demands associated with the [ovum] donation process."[62]

The objections raised by those who question the ethics of compensation for ovum donation generally fall into five broad categories: 1) objections on religious grounds ("selling" eggs is demeaning to women and a wrongful use of reproductive capacity), 2) objections based on the idea that compensation treats ova as commodities, thereby devaluing human life, 3) objections based on the notion that compensation is exploitative and coercive (compensation will create an undue inducement to donate and cause donor's to ignore or discount risks to their own health), 4) objections that view compensation as objectifying children and promoting positive eugenics (recipients may try to buy "super" ova to get offspring with high intelligence or special skills), and 5) objections based on notions of fairness (creating a "market" for ova will lead to higher and higher prices that will eventually make IVF by ovum donation elitist).

---

[61] Ethics Committee of the American Society of Reproductive Medicine, "Financial Incentives in Recruitment of Oocyte Donors," *Fertility and Sterility* August 2000, Vol. 74, No. 2, 218; http://www.asrm.org/Media/Ethics/financial_incentives.pdf.

[62] Ibid. 218-219.

These objections are too numerous and complex to discuss here. Some of them raise legitimate ethical concerns; others are really "red herrings." For example, objections to compensation for ova on religious grounds are really objections to most forms of ART and not to the financial aspects of IVF.[63] All of the legitimate ethical issues can be addressed, in my opinion, by following the recommendations of the Ethics Committee of the American Society of Reproductive Medicine to cap the compensation at a reasonable amount based on the time required to be a donor and risks and discomfort involved, and to avoid paying premiums for special types or classes of donors. Those who want to know more about the ethical issues related to compensation of ovum donors should read the excellent article *Payment for Egg Donation and Surrogacy* by Bonnie Steinbock, Ph.D., Professor and Chair of the Philosophy Department, State University of New York (SUNY) in Albany.[64]

Ethics and Politics

In researching the literature available on the ethical issues raised by compensating donors to sperm banks and ovum donor programs, I was struck by the fact that relatively little has been written about the ethics of men donating sperm for pay while there is a great deal of heated debate about the ethics of compensating ovum donors.

---

[63] See, e.g., "Basic Questions on Sexuality and Reproductive Technology, When is it Right to Intervene?" The Center for Bioethics and Human Dignity, (Kregal Publications, Grand Rapids, MI, 1998) 34. ("[T]he one flesh principle, based on the declaration in Genesis that when a man leaves his family and takes a wife the two become one flesh, . . . allows reproductive technology that enables a husband and wife to produce offspring by assisted means but would exclude the use of donor sperm or eggs being joined with the gametes of the husband or wife.")

[64] Bonnie Steinbock, Ph.D., "Payment for Egg Donation and Surrogacy," The Mount Sinai Journal of Medicine, Sept. 2004: Vol. 71, No.4; http://www.mssm.edu/msjournal/71/71_4_pages_255_265.pdf.

Why is this? I was also struck by the fact that most web sites for ovum donor programs reflect a respectful attitude toward women and recognition that the motives behind the participation of the vast majority of ovum donors are altruistic. By contrast, sperm donor websites often include postings from past or prospective donors that are shockingly profane, crude, and demeaning to women.[65] Why is this? And, more importantly, why has it not drawn critical comment?

The criticism of compensating women for ova—indeed, much of the criticism of women for the exercise of reproductive rights in general—comes primarily from political conservatives. For example, the article referenced above, *Eggheads, Young Women in Need of Cash are Increasingly Deciding to Sell their Bodies*, was written by an editor of the conservative National Review. In deploring the creation of what she calls an "egg market," the author quotes with approval a sociology professor from the City University of New York who comments that "The demand side of the market comes mostly from career-minded baby-boomers, the frontierswomen of feminism, who thought they could have it all."[66]

The stereotyping of women seeking to conceive via ovum donation as "career-minded baby-boomers" and "feminists" rather than seeing them as women of all ages and political philosophies seeking treatment for infertility is characteristic of conservative political dogma. It is reminiscent of the conservative stereotyping of women seeking abortions as either "unmarried teenage girls who have been having sex but have been careless or ignorant in the matter of birth control" or "women who want careers or independent lives and whose deepest aspirations would be destroyed by having a child at this point in their lives." These descriptions are taken from the book *Moral Politics: How Liberals and Conservatives Think*, by cognitive

---

[65] See, e.g., http://www.spermbanker.com/bank/info/top-5-reasons-to-donate-sperm.

[66] Lopez.

linguist George Lakoff.⁶⁷ Lakoff describes these stereotypes as derived from conservative moral categories based on conservative notions of how families should be structured and the proper roles of husbands and wives within families.

It is not my intention to tell others how to answer the tough ethical and moral questions that are raised by ART. But I do want to urge men and women considering using ART to read and listen critically to the various arguments made for and against the use of ART so that they can recognize which arguments are based on science, which on religious philosophy, and which on political stereotypes.

---

⁶⁷ George Lakoff, *Moral Politics: How Liberals and Conservatives Think*, (Chicago: The University of Chicago Press, 2002) 267.

Appendix IV

Avoiding Missteps and Misdirection: Problems with Language

To date, the language and informational materials available to accurately and respectfully reflect the experiences of ART parents simply have *not* been sufficiently developed. In his book, *IVF Children: The First Generation,* Dr. Alastaire Sutcliffe observes: "It is clear . . . that, although we are advising all families to tell their children at a young age about their mode of conception, some are opting not to. This is in part due to a lack of appropriately worded/oriented literature to inform such discussions,"[68]

If you find that the ART books you've read thus far fit nicely into your understanding of infertility and how you see yourself speaking to your children about their origins, then perhaps you will not agree with Dr. Sutcliffe's criticism, but for those ART parents who feel offended by the language recommended by authors who themselves have had no first hand experience raising ART children, I offer the following summary of the problems inherent in the language of the current literature, and I offer alternative language that may more accurately reflect the information they wish to convey.

---

[68] Sutcliffe 109-110.

A well intentioned, but misdirected, example in adult literature can be seen in a series of questions and answers published for ART parents by the American Infertility Association (AIA)[69] in 2000, when there were already an estimated 35,000 ART babies born in that year alone.

A child by donor ovum asks his mother: "What's a genetic parent?"

AIA suggests that the mother answer as follows: "Genes are an important part of the egg, just like they're an important part of the sperm. When the egg and sperm come together and grow, an embryo forms. Genes control traits like the color of our hair or eyes, whether our hair is straight or curly, and how tall we are. Genes determine how we will grow. Some of your genes are from the donor and some are from your father (if this is the case). I am your biological connection to life [note the avoidance of the word "mother" here]—I carried you in my uterus and nurtured you from an embryo into a baby."[70]

What the AIA publication is implying is that when ART involves ovum donation, the father and the *donor* are the child's parents. And the mother, rather than being considered a parent, is described to the child as *"your biological connection to life."* The AIA is, in effect, recommending that the mother tell her child that the donor is the child's genetic mother. But that is totally, outrageously wrong.

Here's my answer to a question that asks about a genetic parent: "A genetic parent is someone who gives a starter cell with some of the genes necessary to help build a baby, and then nurtures and cares for that baby until it is a grown-up and ready to live on its own. But to be parents, mothers and fathers don't have to contribute to all of their baby's genes. Sometimes mothers and fathers need a little help from a genetic donor. That's someone who contributes some genes so that the mother and father can complete making their baby."

---

[69] The American Infertility Association is now called The American Fertility Association (www.theafa.org), a national, nonprofit patient advocacy organization based in New York.

[70] "Talking with Children about Ovum Donation," *The American Infertility Association Fact Sheet,* 19 October 2000.

The AIA's description of genes is also misleading. The quote above suggests that a child gets its traits either from its mother's ovum donor's genes or its father's genes and that these genes combine in the child like some sort of jigsaw puzzle. The truth is, it is *not* a single individual's gene that directs the child's body to have a particular set of blue or brown eyes. It is the new *combination* of genes in the child that determines what physical characteristics are expressed. And the genes that are involved in a characteristic or trait like eye color are exactly the same from person to person throughout the entire family of man.

And let's not forget the nuances of nurture. There is research to support the notion that there may be a significant genetic component to shyness. Yet a trait such as shyness is not inherited as if it were a chunk of personality. Environment is also key. What could be interpreted and responded to as "vulnerable shyness" in one family could be interpreted and responded to in another as "looking before you leap emotionally." In the former instance, the character trait might be perceived as a problem to be "worked on" or corrected. In the latter, the child might be seen as sensitive and wise, characteristics deserving of praise and reinforcement. The child's future sense of self as either "shy" or "sensitive and wise" will also depend on how parents respond to the child's early behaviors. It's a mistake to oversimplify the role of genes in a child's life.

A similar confusion arises when authors, writing from the perspective of the adoption world, try to extrapolate their experience to the world of ART, referring to it as "collaborative reproduction." It may take a village to *raise* a child, but it always takes parents to *create* one. It is *not* fair, accurate, or respectful to tell children that they are the product of a collaborative group effort, no matter how lovingly intended. Every child has the right to enjoy the exclusivity of his family identity and bonding experience.

In their book *Choosing Assisted Reproduction, Social Emotional and Ethical Considerations*, psychologist Susan Cooper and social work counselor Ellen Glazer suggest to parents that "as their child grows older, it is certainly appropriate for parents to acknowledge sadness that their wonderful child did not come from both his parents' genes; that although they would wish for no other child than the one they have, it is a loss for them not to have created him/her together."[71]

I believe this is poor advice to give third party assisted parents for three reasons:

1) It conveys the negative message that something about the child or his origin represents a "loss" to the parents because he "did not come from both his parents' genes."
2) It concludes, erroneously, that the parents didn't "create him/her together," which is as far from the truth as it can be. The parents intentionally and willfully created the child together through their love and the efforts they made that were an expression of that love. The donor did not create the child, leaving out one of the parents in the process. Yet this is the implication: that the donor and one parent created the child, and the other parent played a lesser, non-genetic role in the child's creation.
3) It implies that the parents are sad about a fact of their child's genetic makeup. Nothing could be further from the truth. They were sad and grieving long before the child came into their world. In fact, it is the joy this child brings that allows parents to let go of former sadness. In my opinion, it is inappropriate to project the parental grief of infertility onto a child.

Later, in the same chapter, authors Cooper and Glazer suggest saying to a child: "The donor is your biological (. . . genetic) father (mother) . . . not a parent in a psychological sense, only in a biological sense."

I dislike this wording. Try and explain the distinction between a biological and a psychological parent to a youngster! These authors seem to be presuming that such definitions will somehow provide

---

[71] Susan Cooper and Ellen Glazer, *Choosing Assisted Reproduction, Social Emotional and Ethical Considerations* (Indianapolis: Perspectives Press, 1998) 374.

clarity and comfort to a child. I think such discussions will have the opposite effect, creating unnecessary identity confusion and a sense of loss and guilt. What meaning is the child expected to extract from the adjective "psychological?" Might not such an explanation lead to questions such as: "Is my mommy an incomplete mommy, somehow? Do I have some mysterious other incomplete mommy out there that I have missed, or that I may never know? Maybe I was half-adopted by my mom and dad?"

The point that these authors have missed is that a germ cell donor/contributor is not the same as a genetic parent and never will be. The people who envision, nurture, protect, and love a child are that child's parents, whether they happen to be contributors to the genetic recipe or not. Moreover, these authors misstate the scientific evidence. A biological influence is any influence, genetic or environmental, that can alter the physiology of the developing fetus or child. All pregnant mothers, regardless of genetics, produce numerous neurotransmitters and hormones that cross the placenta to directly impact the expression of genetics in the growing fetus. Non-genetic DE or DI parents exert unique biological influences on their developing child, just as any other parents would.

Recommendations from professionals to ART fathers can also go awry. In her book, *Flight of the Stork, What Children Think about Sex and Family Building*, Dr. Anne Bernstein poses a hypothetical question from a child: "Why didn't the man who gave the sperm for me want to be my daddy?"

Her suggested response: "Your birth father didn't know you and he didn't know me. He gave his sperm to help make babies for people who really wanted babies but couldn't have them without his help. He didn't know who would get his sperm and even if a baby would grow when his sperm was used. He gave his sperm because he wanted to help out, not because he was ready to be a daddy to a child."[72]

---

[72] Anne Bernstein, *Flight of the Stork: What Children Think (and When) about Sex and Family Building* (Indianapolis: Perspectives Press, 1994) 174.

By now, no doubt, you can imagine my view of this. First of all, the sperm donor is not the "birth father." The man who created this child with his wife by seeking out a donor, by supporting his wife during her pregnancy, and by attending the birth is the birth father. Second, many sperm donors are already fine "daddies" to their own children. So why raise an unnecessary fiction about the donor at the end? Also, is it the author's *intention* to distinguish between "fathers" and "daddies?" I see no need to create a fiction in the name of bonding, nor any need to suggest that a daddy is different than a father.

I believe a far better answer to the question would be: "The sperm donor gave his sperm to help mommies *and* daddies who really wanted to make babies *together*. Your origins include the sperm from our donor and mommy's egg, two ingredients of the recipe that mommy and daddy put together so that they could make you."

Again, the distinction should be clear: donors are *never* parents. To try to describe the role of donors, or even gestational carriers, by adding different modifiers to the words "mother," "father," or "parent" is counterproductive, in my opinion.

It is important to note that the psychic importance of genetics will vary from family to family and from child to child. All parents need to be open, attuned, and accepting of whatever interest their child may develop in his or her genetics. But it is inappropriate to *assume* that the role of genetics will be experienced as *the* key factor in children's understanding of their identity. Every child has a right to discover and weigh for him- or herself the meaning of the various elements of genetic contribution, without any pre-programming from well-intentioned counselors using poorly chosen language.

Even in well-written books for young ages that are specifically written for ART parents to share with their children, an important distinction sometimes gets lost about the hierarchy of parents and donors.

In *Mommy, Did I Grow in Your Tummy?* [73] Elaine R. Gordon, Ph.D. writes in clear, comforting language about the many ways

---

[73] Elaine Gordon, *Mommy, Did I Grow in Your Tummy? Where Some Babies Come From* (Santa Monica: EM Greenberg Press, 1992).

children are made, but she fails to make a clear distinction between the role of parents and their donors. In several illustrations in the book, the parents and donor are shown in a format that gives equal weight to all participants. I think such pictures could lead a child to surmise that he/she has three parents and invites confusion where there needn't be any. How much better these illustrations might have been had they been formatted so that the parents are consistently pictured at the top of a hierarchy.

On the other hand, in *Let Me Explain* by Jane T. Schnitter, a book I admire, narrated in the voice of a little girl who was conceived via donor insemination, the language has been carefully crafted to clearly distinguish the parents from the donor. There are no ambiguous qualifiers used with the word "parent" for young readers to ponder, nor is there a false sense of group collaboration to add confusion to the circumstances of the conception. The primary role of the parents is lovingly portrayed throughout the book. The only element of the story that troubles me is the rather simplistic suggestion that genes are accountable for *all* the unique qualities of behavior and appearance that this little girl observes about herself. There is only one brief acknowledgment of the influence of nurturing when the narrator says: "I act like my dad sometimes though, watching football, riding bikes, playing rummy, or saying, 'Oh Baloney!' That's because I've learned these things from him, not because I have his genes on the inside."[74]

In fact, as science tells us, the daughter has not only "learned" such behaviors from her dad, but she's developed specific and receptive neural pathways within her brain as a direct result of the warm relationship she shares with her dad. She has, in effect, incorporated her dad's behaviors into a significant part of her body's neural substance and chemistry.

For any ART parents who read this book with their children, the omission of the role of environment in determining behavior can be explored later when their child is old enough to understand the high school level science of what genes really do and don't do.

---

[74] Jane Schnitter, *Let Me Explain, A Story About Donor Insemination* (Indianapolis: Perspectives Press, 1995) 15.

I don't think it's an accident that Jane Schnitter is one of the few authors who has no difficulty using clear and unambiguous language to distinguish and identify the roles of parents and donors. After all, she is a mother by adoption herself, with two children by birth and eight foster children. As a mom, she obviously understands the importance of language when communicating with children. I wish all authors could be as precise and careful.

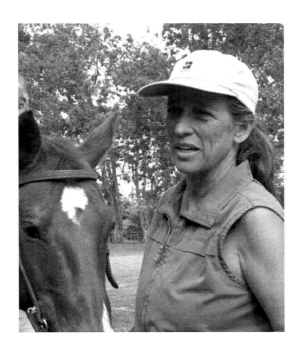

Dr. Lonny Higgins graduated from Wellesley College in 1969 with a BA in Philosophy. She received her MD from Tufts University School of Medicine where she was elected to the Alpha Omega Alpha National Honor Medical Society. She completed her OB/GYN residency at Tufts University and became Board Certified and a Fellow of the American College of Obstetricians and Gynecologists in 1985 after traveling and working in New Zealand and Guam. She lives on her farm on the Big Island of Hawaii with her husband, two of their three children, three horses, 70 sheep, two dogs, and a cat.